HEALTH CARE IN TRANSITION

INDIAN HEALTH CARE

IMPROVEMENT ACT AND HEALTH SERVICE CONSIDERATIONS

Health Care in Transition

Additional books in this series can be found on Nova's website under the Series tab.

Additional E-books in this series can be found on Nova's website under the E-book tab.

Health Care Issues, Costs and Access

Additional books in this series can be found on Nova's website under the Series tab.

Additional E-books in this series can be found on Nova's website under the E-book tab.

HEALTH CARE IN TRANSITION

INDIAN HEALTH CARE

IMPROVEMENT ACT AND HEALTH SERVICE CONSIDERATIONS

JULIUS HANSEN
AND
OLIVER BISHOP
EDITORS

Nova Science Publishers, Inc.
New York

Library of Congress Cataloging-in-Publication Data

ISBN 978-1-61942-323-7

Published by Nova Science Publishers, Inc. † New York

CONTENTS

PREFACE

On March 2010, President Obama signed into law a comprehensive health care reform bill, the Patient Protection and Affordable Care Act (PPACA). The law, among other things, reauthorizes the Indian Health Care Improvement Act (IHCIA) and makes several changes that may affect American Indians and Alaska Natives enrolled in and receiving services from the Medicare, Medicaid, and State Children's Health Insurance Program. This book summarizes some of the key changes made in the reauthorization of IHCIA as it sets out the national policy for health services for Indians.

Chapter 1- On March 23, 2010, President Obama signed into law a comprehensive health care reform bill, the Patient Protection and Affordable Care Act (PPACA; P.L. 111-148). The law, among other things, reauthorizes the Indian Health Care Improvement Act (P.L. 94-3 47, IHCIA), which authorizes many programs and services provided by the Indian Health Service (IHS). In addition, it makes several changes that may affect American Indians and Alaska Natives enrolled in and receiving services from the Medicare, Medicaid, and State Children's Health Insurance Program (CHIP)—also called Social Security Act (SSA) health benefit programs, and it includes changes to private health insurance that may affect American Indians and Alaska Natives and may affect tribes that offer private health insurance.

Chapter 2- On March 23, 2010, President Obama signed into law a comprehensive health care reform bill, the Patient Protection and Affordable Care Act (PPACA; P.L. 111-148). Among its provisions, PPACA reenacts, amends, and permanently reauthorizes the Indian Health Care Improvement Act (IHCIA). IHCIA authorizes many specific Indian Health Service (IHS) activities, sets out the national policy for health services administered to Indians, and sets health condition goals for the IHS service population to reduce "the prevalence and incidence of preventable illnesses among, and unnecessary and premature deaths of, Indians." The reauthorization of IHCIA in PPACA amends the IHCIA to, among other changes, expand programs that seek to augment the IHS health care workforce, increase the amount and type of services available at facilities funded by the IHS, and increase the number and type of programs that provide behavioral health and substance abuse treatment to American Indians and Alaska Natives.

Chapter 3- The Indian Health Service (IHS), an agency in the Department of Health and Human Services (HHS), provides health care to American Indians and Alaska Natives. When care at an IHS-funded facility is unavailable, IHS's contract health services (CHS) program pays for care from external providers if the patient meets certain requirements and funding is available. The Patient Protection and Affordable Care Act requires GAO to study the adequacy of federal funding for IHS's CHS program. To examine program funding needs, IHS collects data on unfunded services—services for which funding was not available—from the federal and tribal CHS programs. GAO examined (1) the extent to which IHS ensures the data it collects on unfunded services are accurate to determine a reliable estimate of CHS program need, (2) the extent to which federal and tribal CHS programs report having funds available to pay for contract health services, and (3) the experiences of external providers in obtaining payment from the CHS program. GAO surveyed 66 federal and 177 tribal CHS programs and spoke to IHS officials and 23 providers.

In: Indian Health Care ISBN: 978-1-61942-323-7
Editors J. Hansen and O. Bishop© 2012 Nova Science Publishers, Inc.

Chapter 1

INDIAN HEALTH CARE: IMPACT OF THE PATIENT PROTECTION AND AFFORDABLE CARE ACT (PPACA)

Elayne J. Heisler

SUMMARY

On March 23, 2010, President Obama signed into law a comprehensive health care reform bill, the Patient Protection and Affordable Care Act (PPACA; P.L. 111-148). The law, among other things, reauthorizes the Indian Health Care Improvement Act (P.L. 94-3 47, IHCIA), which authorizes many programs and services provided by the Indian Health Service (IHS). In addition, it makes several changes that may affect American Indians and Alaska Natives enrolled in and receiving services from the Medicare, Medicaid, and State Children's Health Insurance Program (CHIP)—also called Social Security Act (SSA) health benefit programs, and it includes changes to private health insurance that may affect American Indians and Alaska Natives and may affect tribes that offer private health insurance.

IHCIA authorizes many IHS programs and services, it sets out the national policy for health services administered to Indians, and it articulates the federal goal of ensuring the highest possible health status for Indians, including urban Indians. In addition, it authorizes direct collections from Medicare, Medicaid, and other third-party insurers. Prior to PPACA, IHCIA was last reauthorized in FY2000, although programs have received appropriations since that time. PPACA reauthorizes IHCIA and extends authorizations of appropriations for IHCIA programs indefinitely. It amends a number of sections of IHCIA in general, to permit tribal organizations (TOs) and urban Indian organizations (UIOs) to apply for contract and grant programs for which they were not previously eligible; to create new mental health prevention and treatment programs, including new youth suicide prevention programs; and to require demonstration projects to construct modular and mobile health facilities in order to expand health services available through IHS, Indian Tribes (ITs), and TOs. It also made several organizational changes to IHS. It requires IHS to establish an Office of Direct Service Tribes to serve tribes that receive their health care and other services directly from IHS as opposed to receiving services through IHS-funded facilities or programs operated by ITs or TOs. In addition, the law requires IHS to develop a plan to establish a new area office to serve tribes in Nevada and requires the Secretary of the Department of Health and Human Services (HHS) to appoint a new IHS Director of HIV/AIDS Prevention and Treatment.

In addition to reauthorizing IHCIA, PPACA includes a number of provisions that may affect American Indians and Alaska Natives who receive services through SSA health benefit programs or who have private insurance coverage. With regard to SSA health benefit programs, the new law permits specified Indian entities to determine Medicaid and CHIP eligibility and extends the period during which IHS, IT, and TO services are reimbursed for all Medicare Part B services, indefinitely, beginning January 1, 2010. Prior to PPACA, authority for these facilities to receive Medicare Part B reimbursements for certain specified services had expired on January 1, 2010. With regard to private insurance coverage, PPACA provides a special enrollment period for American Indians and Alaska Natives who may enroll in private insurance offered through an exchange and excludes tribal health benefits from being counted as gross income for tax purposes.

INTRODUCTION

On March 23, 2010, President Obama signed into law a comprehensive health care reform bill, the Patient Protection and Affordable Care Act (PPACA; P.L. 111-148), which, among other things, reauthorizes the Indian Health Care Improvement Act (P.L. 94-347, IHCIA). This report, one of a series of CRS products on PPACA, summarizes some of the key changes made in the reauthorization of IHCIA. In addition, the report summarizes other PPACA provisions related to American Indians and Alaska Natives enrolled in and receiving services from Medicare, Medicaid, and the State Children's Health Insurance Program (CHIP)—also called SSA health benefit programs[1] and changes to private health insurance coverage that may affect American Indians and Alaska Natives enrolled in or Indian tribes that offer private health insurance.

The report begins with an overview of the Indian Health Service (IHS) and IHCIA. It then discusses each of the eight titles in IHCIA and how PPACA amends each of these titles. Finally, the report discusses other PPACA changes that may affect American Indians and Alaska Natives. For each topic, including each IHCIA title, discussed, the report first gives a brief description for context, and then describes the changes made by PPACA.

OVERVIEW OF INDIAN HEALTH CARE

The Indian Health Service (IHS), an agency within the Department of Health and Human Services (HHS), provides health care for approximately 1.9 million eligible American Indians/Alaska Natives through a system of programs and facilities located on or near Indian reservations, and through contractors in certain urban areas.[2] IHS provides services in 35 states, subdivided into 12 geographic "Areas" that consist of one or more states.[3] Each Area is administered by an Area Office; Areas, in turn, are further subdivided into service units that consist of one or more facilities. IHS may provide services directly, or Indian tribes (ITs) or tribal organizations (TOs) may operate IHS facilities and programs themselves through self-determination contracts and self-governance compacts negotiated with IHS.[4] Although most IHS facilities are located on or near reservations, IHS also funds urban Indian health projects (UIHPs), through grants or contracts to urban Indian organizations (UIOs).

The IHS provides an array of medical services, including inpatient, ambulatory, emergency, dental, public health nursing, and preventive health care.[5] The IHS does not have a defined medical benefit package that excludes or includes specific conditions or types of health care. Besides providing general clinical health services, the IHS also focuses on health conditions prevalent among American Indians and Alaska Natives such as infant mortality, diabetes, and hepatitis B. In addition, IHS provides mental health and alcohol and substance abuse services because, compared to the overall

U.S. population, American Indians and Alaska Natives are more likely to die from alcoholism-related diseases or to commit suicide.[6]

In addition to health services, the IHS funds projects related to health care facilities and sanitation. Specifically, the IHS funds the construction, equipping, and maintenance of hospitals, health centers, clinics, and other health care delivery facilities, both those operated by the IHS and those operated by tribes. In order to improve the health of, and reduce the incidence of disease among, American Indians and Alaska Natives, the IHS also funds the construction of water supply and sewage facilities and solid waste disposal systems, and provides technical assistance for the operation and maintenance of such facilities. The IHS has attributed decreases in gastrointestinal disease among American Indians and Alaska Natives to improved sanitation facilities.[7]

Indian Health Care Improvement Act

The Indian Health Care Improvement Act, as passed in 1976 and subsequently amended, authorized many specific IHS activities,[8] set out the national policy for health services administered to Indians, and declared that it was a federal goal to improve the health status and conditions of the IHS service population. IHCIA also authorized direct collections from Medicare, Medicaid, and other third-party insurers for American Indians and Alaska Natives receiving services at facilities operated by the IHS, an IT, or a TO. IHCIA gave IHS authority to grant funding to UIOs to provide health care services to urban Indians, and established substance abuse treatment programs, Indian health professions recruitment programs, and many other programs. Prior to PPACA, IHCIA was last fully reauthorized by the Indian Health Amendments of 1992,[9] which extended authorizations of its appropriations through FY2000. In 2000, all IHCIA authorizations of appropriations were extended through FY2001.[10] Congress has continued to appropriate funds for IHCIA programs since 2001.[11] IHCIA reauthorization had been under consideration in Congress since 1999.[12]

IHCIA Reauthorization in PPACA

Title X, "Strengthening Quality, Affordable Health Care for All Americans," of PPACA in Subtitle B, "Provisions Relating to Title II," Part III, amends and enacts the "Indian Health Care Improvement Reauthorization and Extension Act of 2009 (S. 1790)," as reported by the Senate Committee on Indian Affairs on December 16, 2009.[13] In addition, Title II, "Role of Public Programs," Subtitle K, "Protections for American Indians and Alaska Natives," contains provisions related to American Indians and Alaska Natives in SSA health benefit programs and in the private health insurance exchange established by PPACA.[14] PPACA reauthorizes IHCIA permanently and indefinitely; it appropriates such sums as may be necessary for FY20 10 and each fiscal year thereafter, to remain available until expended. PPACA maintains IHCIA's eight Titles but amends and adds a number of sections to each of the titles. Table 1 summarizes the changes that PPACA makes to IHCIA.

Table 1. IHCIA Reauthorization Summary

Title Name and Subject	PPACA
Title I-Indian Health Manpower Authorizes workforce programs to increase the supply of providers at IHS facilities	Maintains title's major sections; repeals section authorizing appropriations for the title; expands use of community health aide workers at IHS-funded facilities; adds a new section funding a demonstration to address IHS health professional shortages; and exempts employees at IHS-funded facilities from certain licensing, registration requirements and related fees.
Title II-Health Services Authorizes IHS health services, research, payments for service-related transportation, payment for services provided through contracts with outside providers (i.e., Contract Health Services (CHS))	Maintains title's major sections; repeals section authorizing appropriations for the title; amends authorization for 2 funds (Indian Health Care Improvement Fund and Catastrophic Health Emergency Fund); expands IHS authority for diabetes, cancer screening, and long-term care programs; and amends sections related to the CHS program.
Title III-Health Facilities Authorizes construction and renovation of IHS facilities; sets procedures by which construction and renovation projects are selected	Maintains title's major sections; repeals section authorizing appropriations for the title; amends IHS construction priority system; and adds new sections requiring grants to build modular and mobile facilities.
Title IV-Access to Health Services	Maintains title's major sections; repeals section authorizing appropriations for the

Table 1. (Continued)

Title Name and Subject	PPACA
Authorizes IHS programs to bill Medicare, Medicaid, and private insurance	title; adds the State Children's Health Insurance Program to programs that IHS is authorized to bill; adds new sections permitting ITs, TOs, and UIOS to purchase federal employee health and life insurance benefits for their employees; expands IHS collaboration with the Department of Veterans Affairs and the Department of Defense.
Title V-Health Services for Urban Indians Authorizes grants to UIOs for health projects to serve urban Indians	Maintains title's major sections; repeals section authorizing appropriations for the title; expands grant opportunities available to UIOs.
Title VI-Organization Improvements Establishes IHS's organizational position within HHS; the position of Director of IHS; and requires an automated management information system for IHS record-keeping	Maintains title's major sections; establishes that the IHS Director should report directly to the HHS Secretary; adds new sections requiring: (1) an Office of Direct Service Tribes; and (2) a plan to create a new Nevada Area Office.
Title VII-Behavioral Health Programs Authorizes programs related to behavioral health prevention and treatment	Replaces IHCIA Title VII with new language authorizing new comprehensive behavioral health and treatment programs. Includes a new subsection authorizing programs related to youth suicide prevention.
Title VIII-Miscellaneous Requires the IHS Director to submit a number of reports; establishes IHS eligibility for health services; and defines California Indians, amongst other provisions	Maintains title's major sections; repeals section authorizing appropriations for the title; adds new sections that, among other things, establish: (1) a prescription drugs monitoring program; (2) an IHS Director of HIV/AIDS Prevention and Treatment; and (3) new requirements for the IHS budget requests to reflect inflation and changes in the IHS service population.

Source: CRS analysis of P.L. 94-437, as amended (IHCIA), and P.L. 111-148 (PPACA).

Definitions

PPACA defines a number of new Indian-related terms. Two of the new terms most frequently used are Indian Health Program and Tribal Health Program. "Indian Health Program" (IHP) is defined as (1) any health program administered by the IHS, (2) any Tribal Health Program, or (3) any Indian tribe or tribal organization to which the Secretary provides funding under the Buy Indian Act. "Tribal Health Program" (THP) is defined as any IT or TO operating any health program, service, function, activity, or facility funded, in whole or part, by the IHS through, or provided for in, a contract or compact with the IHS under the Indian Self-Determination and Education Assistance Act (ISDEAA). In addition, the bill maintains a number of IHCIA-defined terms.

Selected Major Changes

Purposes and Findings: PPACA adds a new finding that articulates that it is a major national goal of the United States to provide resources, processes, and structure that will enable ITs and tribal members to obtain the quantity and quality of health care services and opportunities that will eradicate health disparities between Indians and the general population.

Appropriations: PPACA consolidates authorizations of appropriations into a single provision, authorizes such sums as may be necessary, and extends authorizations of appropriations indefinitely. In addition, PPACA repeals the separate authorizations of appropriations that had been included at the end of each IHCIA title or had been included in specific IHCIA sections.

Expanded Access to UIOs and TOs: PPACA permits TOs and UIOs to apply for grant and contract programs for which these entities were previously not eligible.

Behavioral Health Programs: PPACA expands mental health services to create a comprehensive behavioral health and treatment program. It includes programs related to youth suicide prevention and increases IT and TO access to grants sponsored by the Substance Abuse and Mental Health Services Administration (SAMHSA).

Payor of Last Resort: PPACA states that IHS is the payor of last resort for all services provided. Under current regulations,[15] IHS is the payor of last resort only for contract health services (CHS)—services that IHS, ITs, or TOs may purchase, through contracts, from private providers in instances where the IHP cannot provide the needed care.

Indians in SSA Programs: PPACA extends Medicare payments to hospitals operated by IHS, ITs, or TOs, and permits Indian entities to determine Medicaid and CHIP eligibility in order to facilitate American Indian and Alaska Native enrollment in Medicaid and CHIP.

Office of Direct Service Tribes: PPACA requires that IHS establish an Office of Direct Service Tribes to serve tribes that receive their health care and other services directly from IHS rather than through facilities or programs operated by ITs or TOs.

Nevada Area Office: PPACA requires a plan to establish a new area office to serve tribes in Nevada.

Demonstration Projects: PPACA includes two facilities demonstration projects that will award funds for IHS, ITs, or TOs to construct modular and mobile health facilities.

Title I: Indian Health, Human Resources, and Development

IHCIA Title I included provisions related to increasing the number of American Indians and Alaska Natives entering the health professions in order to increase the supply of health professionals available to facilities and programs operated by IHS, ITs, and TOs. The IHS has high vacancy rates in many of its health professions—over 20% for physicians, and over 15% for dentists, and nurses, for instance, as of December 2009.[16] IHCIA authorized a number of workforce programs, including, for example, scholarship and loan repayment programs, to encourage health professionals to work at facilities operated by the IHS or ITs; funding for continuing education for IHS employees; funding for advanced training and for recruitment and retention for individuals working at facilities operated by the IHS, an IT, a TO, or a UIO;

training for nursing; and programs to encourage American Indians and Alaska Natives to enter medicine. In addition, Title I authorized two innovative health professions programs: the community health representative (CHR) program, which permits the training of American Indians and Alaska Natives to serve as paraprofessionals who provide health care, health promotion, and disease prevention services at IHS facilities; and the community health aide program (CHAP), which provides training for Alaska Natives to serve as health aides or community health practitioners.

PPACA maintains and reauthorizes a number of these health professions programs. It expands the CHAP program to areas outside of Alaska, but excludes CHAP's dental health aide therapist program in Alaska from states outside of Alaska unless an IT or a TO, in a state authorizing such a program, elects to include it. PPACA also includes additional requirements for the Secretary to facilitate the implementation of the CHAP dental health aide program by ITs and TOs and prohibits the Secretary from filling IHS program vacancies for certified dentists with dental health aide therapists.

TITLE II: HEALTH SERVICES

IHCIA Title II authorized a number of specific health programs and activities, including mental health programs, prevention activities, diabetes and tuberculosis programs, Indian women's health, Indian school health education programs, epidemiological centers, and a fund for the elimination of backlogs and deficiencies among Indian health programs (called the Indian Health Care Improvement Fund (IHCIF)), and other programs. The title also included provisions relating to CHS delivery areas in several states.[17] CHS services are limited to American Indians and Alaska Natives living in defined geographic areas called CHS delivery areas.

PPACA reauthorizes the IHCIF as well as the Catastrophic Health Emergency Fund (which provides extra funding to facilities with extraordinary medical costs because of disasters and catastrophic illnesses). It expands the range of health promotion and disease prevention activities required to be provided, and includes new authorizations for hospice care, assisted living, longterm care, and home- and community-based services for disabled elderly persons. Title II also expands the Indians into Psychology Program, the Indian youth grant program, epidemiology centers, prevention and control of communicable and infectious diseases, requirements for prompt IHS payments to CHS providers, and timely notification to providers that CHS patients are exempt from payment for CHS services.

PPACA also requires the Secretary to maintain any existing or future model diabetes projects, and requires recurring funding for THPs' model diabetes projects.

TITLE III: FACILITIES

IHCIA Title III includes provisions related to health care and sanitation facilities. IHS funds the construction, equipping, and maintenance of hospitals, health centers, clinics, and other health care delivery facilities for facilities operated by IHS and tribes. IHS also funds the construction of sanitation facilities, including water-supply and sewage facilities and solid waste disposal systems, and provides technical assistance for the operation and maintenance of such facilities. IHCIA required the Secretary to ensure that pay rates on such facility construction or renovation projects, if funded under IHCIA Title III, must not fall below the prevailing local wage rates, as determined in accordance with the Davis-Bacon Act.[18]

PPACA maintains current pay rate requirements; it requires the development of a priority system for construction of Indian health care facilities, with a methodology to be reported to Congress, and with priority lists for the 10 highest-priority facilities in five categories of facilities (inpatient, outpatient, specialized facilities, staff quarters, and facility-related hostels). The priority system also permits new facilities to be nominated at least every three years, but protects the priority of facilities at the top of the current lists for construction. The law also requires consultation with ITs and TOs to develop innovative approaches to solving unmet healthcare facility needs, and includes an "area distribution fund" as an option for such innovation. Under the concept of an area distribution fund, each IHS area would receive at least some health facilities construction funding, which was not the case prior to IHCIA reauthorization.

PPACA creates a facilities needs assessment workgroup and a facilities appropriations advisory board in IHS. It maintains authorization for construction of sanitation and water-supply facilities, requires reports to Congress on the priority system for such facilities, authorizes the Secretary to accept major renovations or modernizations of Indian health facilities carried out by ITs, and requires grants to ITs and TOs for construction or upgrading of small ambulatory care facilities.

PPACA also includes a new provision that authorizes the Secretary to accept funding from any other source for facilities construction. It explicitly authorizes other federal agencies to transfer funds, equipment, or supplies to the Secretary for facilities construction and related activities, makes sanitation as well as health care facilities eligible, requires the Secretary to establish health and sanitation facility construction standards by regulation, and specifies that the Secretary's receipt of funds from other sources would not affect priorities established under Section 301 of IHCIA Title III. In addition, PPACA authorizes a new demonstration grant program for modular component health care facilities in Indian communities, and a new demonstration program for mobile health stations for providing specialty health care services.

TITLE IV: ACCESS TO HEALTH SERVICES

IHCIA Title IV contained sections related to billing, and enrollment in, the Medicare and Medicaid programs operated by the Centers for Medicare and Medicaid Services (CMS);[19] a section authorizing appropriations; and a section that authorized emergency CHS services. The title's authorization for IHS health care facilities to receive reimbursements from the Medicare and Medicaid program was a major component of the original IHCIA passed in 1976. Prior to PPACA, IHCIA did not mention funds received under the Children's Health Insurance (CHIP) program because the program was enacted after IHCIA was last reauthorized.[20]

Title IV contained provisions related to billing and receiving reimbursements from the Medicare and Medicaid programs. Specifically, IHCIA: (1) authorized a demonstration project that permits ITs or TOs operating under ISDEAA contracts or compacts to directly bill CMS for Medicare and Medicaid payments; (2) required direct billing reimbursements be placed into a "special fund" that must be used first to achieve compliance with Medicare and Medicaid requirements and then, if excess funds exist, to improve health services available to the population the facility serves; (3) specified the auditing and other requirements related to direct billing; and (4) required that the federal government pay 100% of the cost of all Medicaid services billed.[21] In addition, IHCIA required that reimbursements from Medicare or Medicaid may not be considered when determining annual Indian health appropriations, required the Secretary to submit a report accounting for

Medicare and Medicaid funds reimbursed to IHS, and required the Secretary to make grants to ITs or TOs to facilitate enrollment in Medicare and Medicaid.

PPACA maintains SSA health benefit reimbursement requirements, but adds reimbursements received from the CHIP program to these requirements. For example, reimbursements received from CHIP are included in the requirement that reimbursements from SSA health benefit programs not be taken into account when determining IHS appropriations. PPACA also expands and makes permanent the prior demonstration project that permitted ITs or TOs operating under ISDEAA contracts or compacts to directly bill CMS for Medicare and Medicaid payments and excludes such direct billing reimbursements from the special fund. PPACA also includes grants for outreach and enrollment into SSA health benefit programs and maintains and expands current authorization to recover reimbursements from third-party entities and to credit such reimbursements to the facility that provided the services. In addition, PPACA authorizes ITs, TOs, and UIOs to use SSA health benefit funds and ISDEAA funds to purchase health care coverage and permits ITs, TOs, and UIOs to purchase Federal Employee Health Benefits and Federal Employee Group Life Insurance coverage for their employees. PPACA requires that federal health care programs accept an entity operated by the IHS, an IT, a TO, or a UIO as a provider eligible to receive payments, on the same basis as other qualified providers, if it meets the applicable licensure requirements for its provider type, regardless of whether the facility obtains the applicable license. PPACA also applies this licensing requirement to providers working at Indian entities, and prohibits providers and entities that are excluded from receiving reimbursements from other federal programs from receiving reimbursements from Indian entities.

PPACA also expands IHS 's relationship with the Department of Veterans Affairs (VA) and the Department of Defense (DOD) by authorizing increased coordination to treat Indian veterans. In addition, PPACA requires the Secretary to conduct a study to determine the feasibility of treating the Navajo Nation as a state for Medicaid purposes, for Indians living within the Navajo Nation's boundaries.[22]

TITLE V: HEALTH SERVICES FOR URBAN INDIANS

IHCIA Title V directed the HHS Secretary to make contracts with or grants to UIOs for health projects to serve urban Indians, and set requirements for the contracts and grants. Such grants or contracts are under the authority of the Snyder Act,[23] not the ISDEAA. The purpose of Title V programs is to make health services more accessible and available to urban Indians. Urban Indian Health Projects (UIHPs) may serve a wider range of eligible persons than the general IHS health care programs, including not only members of federally recognized tribes but also members of terminated[24] or state-recognized tribes, as well as their children and grandchildren.

Currently there are 34 UIHPs operating at 41 locations, with different programs offering different services, such as ambulatory health care, health promotion and education, immunizations, case management, child abuse prevention and treatment, and behavioral health services.[25] Besides IHS grants and contracts, UIHPs receive funding from state and private sources, patient fees,[26] Medicaid, Medicare, and other non-IHS federal programs.[27]

PPACA enables UIOs to expand their urban Indian health programs by permitting UIOs to establish a UIHP in urban centers other than where the UIO is located; prior to PPACA UIOs could only establish UIHPs in the urban area where the UIO was based. In addition, PPACA provides UIOs access to goods and services purchased through federal prime vendors, by deeming UIOs with Title V contracts or grants to be federal executive agencies under the section of the Federal Property and Administrative Services Act of 1974[28] concerning federal sources of supply. It also authorizes the Secretary to donate excess or surplus property to such UIOs and to permit the UIOs to use HHS facilities. PPACA also expands to UIOs the authorization for a number of programs currently only at IHS, IT, or TO facilities. For example, PPACA authorizes UIOs to employ Community Health Representatives (CHRs) trained under the CHR program authorized under current IHCIA Title I, and authorizes the Secretary to establish programs for UIOs that are identical to IHS programs for prevention of communicable diseases, for behavioral health prevention and treatment, and for youth multi-drug abuse prevention and treatment. PPACA also authorizes grants to UIOs for the development and implementation of health information technology, telemedicine, and related infrastructure.

TITLE VI: ORGANIZATIONAL IMPROVEMENTS

IHCIA Title VI established IHS as part of the Public Health Service (PHS) within HHS, and is administered by a Director who reports to the HHS Assistant Secretary for Health. IHCIA Title VI also required the Secretary to establish an automated management information system for IHS and IHPs, with a patient privacy component, and requires that patients have access to their own IHS records.

PPACA maintains the placement of IHS in PHS, but directs the head of IHS to report directly to the HHS Secretary. It also maintains requirements regarding the automated management information system. PPACA also adds two new requirements: the Secretary must establish an IHS Office of Direct Service Tribes (for tribes served directly by IHS instead of under ISDEAA), and the Secretary must submit to Congress a plan to create a new Nevada Area Office (Nevada is currently within the Phoenix Area Office).

TITLE VII: BEHAVIORAL HEALTH PROGRAMS

IHCIA Title VII authorized alcohol and substance abuse programs, including grant and contract programs to provide comprehensive alcohol and substance abuse prevention and treatment services. It required coordination with the Department of the Interior to assess the need for such services and to provide community education in alcohol and substance abuse; requires services to specified groups including women and youth; and authorizes training and community education programs, demonstration projects to establish substance abuse counseling education curricula at tribally operated community colleges, and grants for preventing, treating, and diagnosing fetal alcohol syndrome (FAS) and fetal alcohol effects. In addition, Title VII included authorization for substance abuse treatment projects in specified locations in New Mexico, Arizona, and Alaska.

PPACA replaces current IHCIA Title VII with new language that authorizes programs to create a "comprehensive behavioral health prevention and treatment program" providing a "continuum of behavioral health care." For example, PPACA includes programs related to behavioral health prevention and treatment; provisions related to training and licensure requirements for the behavioral health workforce serving at facilities operated by IHS, ITs, or TOs; specific programs to treat Indian women and youth; and programs to treat and prevent child sexual abuse and fetal alcohol disorder. Many of these programs are similar to those that were authorized in IHCIA Title VII. PPACA also includes a new program to award grants to ITs and TOs to carry out demonstration projects using telehealth technology to provide youth suicide prevention and treatment services and authorizes appropriations of $1.5 million for each of FY2010-FY2013 for the new program. In addition, PPACA includes authorization for programs to prevent and treat domestic and sexual violence, and includes a number of requirements for the Secretary to facilitate ITs' and TOs' applying for, and inclusion in, grants from SAMHSA. It also requires the Secretary to carry out activities to increase the use of pre-doctoral psychology and psychiatry interns in order to increase access to mental health services, and authorizes the Secretary to establish a demonstration program through SAMSHA to test a culturally appropriate life skills curriculum to prevent suicide in American Indian and Alaska Native adolescents. PPACA also authorizes an appropriation of $1 million for each of FY2010-FY2014 for the Secretary to establish a grant program to award grants to ITs, TOs, or other entities to establish life skills curriculums to prevent suicide in schools located in high suicide areas that serve Indian children.

TITLE VIII: MISCELLANEOUS

IHCIA Title VIII included a number of separate provisions covering reports, regulations, an IHCIA implementation plan, abortion, eligibility for IHS services, service unit funding reductions, and a variety of other topics.

PPACA maintains a number of IHCIA requirements including those requiring reports, regulations, an IHCIA implementation plan, and those defining individuals eligible for IHS services. PPACA extends the prior IHCIA limitation on the use of federal funds for abortions to IHS, and applies restrictions contained in other federal laws to IHS appropriations. PPACA also makes IHP and UIO medical quality assurance records confidential, and adds several new required reports. PPACA requires a new report on disease and injury prevention, and two new Government Accountability Office reports: (1) on the coordination of Indian health care services provided through IHS, Medicare, Medicaid, or CHIP, or with tribal, state, or local funds; and (2) on the CHS program, including CHS payments to providers (since CHS providers still experience late payments).

PPACA also requires that IHS budget requests reflect inflation and changes in the IHS service population, and requires the establishment of a prescription drug monitoring program at IHP and UIO facilities. PPACA also permits a tribe operating an IHS health program through an ISDEAA self-governance compact to charge Indians for services; adds language stating that the United States has no liability for injury or death resulting from traditional health care practices; and establishes an IHS Director of HIV/AIDS Prevention and Treatment.

Other Provisions

PPACA also includes the reauthorization of the Native Hawaiian Health Care Act of 1988,[29] which authorizes health education, health promotion, disease prevention services, and health professions scholarship programs for Native Hawaiians.[30] It extends the act's authorizations of appropriations through FY20 19, permits a specified school in Hawaii to offer educational programs to Native Hawaiians first, and amends a definition in the act.[31] PPACA also includes provisions related to American Indians and Alaska Natives the individual mandate and the Health Insurance Exchange established in Title I of PPACA. Specifically, Sec. 1311(c)(6)(d) requires a special Exchange enrollment period for American Indians and Alaska Natives; Sec. 1411(b)(5)(A) permits American Indians and Alaska Natives who meet the definition of "Indian" in ISDEAA to seek an exemption from the individual mandate; and Sec. 1501 exempts members of Indian tribes from any penalty associated with a failure to comply with the individual mandate.[32] In addition, Sec. 9021 excludes the value of Indian tribe health benefits from calculations of gross income for tax purposes.[33]

SSA Health Benefit Improvements for Indians

PPACA amends the SSA to define a number of Indian terms as they are defined in IHCIA Section 4. These terms include IHS, IT, TOs, UIOs, IHPs, and THPs. These definitions apply for Medicare, Medicaid, and CHIP and general provisions included in SSA Title XI.

PPACA includes amendments to the SSA, although these amendments are not included in the "Indian Health Care Improvement" part of the bill. Rather, amendments to the SSA are included in Title II, Subtitle K, "Protections for American Indians and Alaska Natives." This subtitle does the following: (1) it designates facilities operated by IHS, an IT, a TO, or a UIO as the payor of last resort notwithstanding federal or state law to the contrary;[34] (2) it includes IHS, ITs, and TOs as entities that are permitted to determine Medicaid and CHIP eligibility; (3) it prohibits cost sharing for Indians whose incomes are at or below 300% of the federal poverty level and who are enrolled in a qualified health benefit plan in the individual market through the exchange (as established by PPACA);[35] and (4) it extends the period for which IHS, IT, and TO services are reimbursed by Medicare Part B for all services, indefinitely, beginning January 1, 2010. Prior to PPACA, authority for these facilities to receive Medicare Part B reimbursements for certain specified services had expired on January 1, 2010. In addition, PPACA, in Title III, amended the Medicare Part D program to permit costs paid by IHS for prescription drugs for Medicare Part D beneficiaries to count toward the beneficiaries' out-of-pocket threshold for catastrophic protection. In order for a Part D beneficiary to receive catastrophic protection, a certain level of out-of-pocket costs must be incurred; prior to PPACA, expenses incurred by IHS, on behalf of a Part D beneficiary, did not count toward this threshold.[36]

End Notes

[1] Other provisions in PPACA may also affect Indian health. For example, Indian tribes may be eligible for new grant or contract programs that augment the health care workforce or improve public health, they may participate in reforms made to the private insurance market, and they may benefit from Medicare and Medicaid reforms. More information about PPACA changes can be found at CRS's website under "Issue in Focus-Health Reform" at http://www.crs.gov/ Pages/subissue.aspx?cliid=3746&parentid=13.

[2] U.S. Department of Health and Human Services, Indian Health Service, IHS Fact Sheet: IHS Year 2010 Profile http://info.ihs.gov/Profile2010.asp.

[3] IHS provides services to American Indians and Alaska Natives residing in 35 states. Area offices may serve tribes in one state, such as the Alaska Area office that administers services in Alaska, or may serve tribes in multiple states, such as the Nashville Area office that administers services for tribes on the east coast, in Alabama, Louisiana, and parts of Texas.

[4] Authorized by P.L. 93-638, the Indian Self-Determination and Education Assistance Act of January 4, 1975, 88 Stat. 2203, as amended; 25 U.S.C. 450 et seq.

[5] See 42 CFR 136.11, "Services available."

[6] IHS, *Trends in Indian Health, 2002-2003*, Part 4: General Mortality Statistics.

[7] U.S. Department of Health and Human Services, Indian Health Service, "IHS Fact Sheets: Safe Water and Waste Disposal Facilities," press release, January 2010, http://info.ihs.gov/Safe Water.asp.

[8] In addition to IHCIA, the Snyder Act of 1921 (P.L. 67-85, act of November 2, 1921, 42 Stat. 208, as amended; 25 U.S.C. 13) also authorizes Indian health programs.

[9] P.L. 102-573, act of October 29, 1992, 106 Stat. 4526.

[10] Omnibus Indian Advancement Act, P.L. 106-568, § 815, act of December 27, 2000, 114 Stat. 2868, 2918.

[11] For a discussion of the relationship between appropriations and authorizations, see CRS Report RS20371, *Overview of the Authorization-Appropriations Process*, by Bill Heniff Jr.

[12] IHCIA reauthorization bills were introduced in the 106th (H.R. 3397 and S. 2526), 107th (S. 212 and H.R. 1662), 108th (S. 556 and H.R. 2440), 109th (H.R. 5312, S. 1057, S. 3524, and S. 4122), 110th (H.R. 1328, S. 1200, and S. 2532); and 111th (H.R. 2708 and S. 1790) Congresses.

[13] This is S. 1790 in 111th Congress.

[14] More information about the private health insurance provisions in PPACA can be found in CRS Report R40942, *Private Health Insurance Provisions in the Patient Protection and Affordable Care Act (PPACA)*, by Hinda Chaikind, Bernadette Fernandez, and Mark Newsom. In addition, PPACA contains other changes that may affect American Indians and

Alaska Natives, but these are not discussed in this report. For Medicare-related changes, see CRS Report R41 196, *Medicare Provisions in the Patient Protection and Affordable Care Act (PPACA): Summary and Timeline*, coordinated by Patricia A. Davis. For information on Medicaid and Children's Health Insurance Program-related provisions, CRS Report R41210, *Medicaid and the State Children's Health Insurance Program (CHIP) Provisions in PPACA: Summary and Timeline*, coordinated by Julie Stone For public health, workforce, and quality-related changes, see CRS Report R41278, *Public Health, Workforce, Quality, and Related Provisions in PPACA: Summary and Timeline*, coordinated by C. Stephen Redhead and Erin D. Williams.

[15] See 42 C.F.R.136.61.

[16] U.S. Department of Health and Human Services, Public Health Service, Indian Health Service, *Indian Health Service: Fiscal Year 2011 Justification of Estimates for Appropriations Committees* (Rockville, MD: HHS/PHS/IHS, 2009); http://www.ihs.gov/NonMedical Programs/BudgetFormulation/documents/IHS%20FY%202011%20Congressional%20 Justification.pdf.

[17] These states are Arizona, California, North Dakota, and South Dakota.

[18] Act of March 3, 1931, chap. 411, 71st Cong., 46 Stat. 1494, as amended; 40 U.S.C., Chap. 31, Subchap. IV. The Davis-Bacon Act requires that employers pay prevailing wage rates, as determined by the Secretary of Labor, on federal construction projects. For more information, see CRS Report R41469, *Davis-Bacon Prevailing Wages and State Revolving Loan Programs Under the Clean Water Act and the Safe Drinking Water Act*, by Gerald Mayer and Jon O. Shimabukuro.

[19] CMS programs are also referred to herein as SSA health benefits programs.

[20] See CRS Report R40444, *State Children's Health Insurance Program (CHIP): A Brief Overview*, by Elicia J. Herz and Evelyne P. Baumrucker.

[21] In general, Medicaid is a shared federal and state program in which the state government pays a share of Medicaid expenses based on a formula where the federal share is inversely proportional to the state's per capita income (i.e., states with lower per capita income receive a greater percentage of Medicaid payments from the federal government).

[22] The Navajo reservation is located in parts of Arizona, Utah, and New Mexico.

[23] The Snyder Act of 1921 (P.L. 67-85, act of November 2, 1921, 42 Stat. 208, as amended; 25 U.S.C. 13) provides general authorization for Indian health programs. The Snyder Act is a permanent, indefinite authorization for federal Indian programs, including for "conservation of health."

[24] "Terminated" tribes are tribes whose federal recognition was withdrawn by statute.

[25] U.S. Department of Health and Human Services, Public Health Service, Indian Health Service, *Indian Health Service: Fiscal Year 2010 Justification of Estimates for Appropriations Committees* (Rockville, MD: HHS/PHS/IHS, 2009), p. CJ-133; http://www.ihs.gov/Non MedicalPrograms/BudgetFormulation/documents/IHS_CJ_2010_Final_Submission.pdf.

[26] IHS is forbidden to bill or charge Indians (see 25 U.S.C. 1681 and 25 USC 458aaa-14), but IHCIA, Title V does not prohibit UIHPs from charging their patients.

[27] IHS, Office of Urban Indian Health Programs, *Urban Indian Health Program Statistics, FY2005* (Rockville, MD: October 16, 2007), p. 4.

[28] Sec. 201(a), P.L. 81-152, act of June 30, 1949, 63 Stat. 377, 383, as amended; 40 U.S.C. 501.

[29] P.L. 100-579, act of October 31, 1988, 102 Stat. 2916, as amended; 42 U.S.C., Chap 122 (§11701 et seq.).

[30] This program receives appropriations through the federal health center program. For more information, see http://bphc.hrsa.gov/about/specialpopulations.htm.

[31] For details, see *The Indian Health Care Improvement Act Reauthorization and Extension Act of 2009 as Enacted by PPACA: Detailed Summary and Timeline by Elayne J. Heisler.*

[32] CRS Report R4133 1, *Individual Mandate and Related Information Requirements under PPA CA* , by Hinda Chaikind.

[33] Section 9021 excludes the following health benefits from calculations of gross income: (1) health services or benefits provided or purchased by IHS, an IT, or a TO or through programs of third parties funded by the IHS; (2) medical care services, including those provided, purchased, or reimbursed by an IT or TO or to a member of an IT and the member's spouse or dependents; (3) accident or health plan coverage (or an arrangement having the same effect) provided by an IT or TO for medical care to a member of an IT and the member's spouse or dependents; and (4) any other medical care provided by an IT that supplements, replaces, or substitutes for the programs and services provided by the federal government to IT or tribal members.

[34] Prior to PPACA, IHS was the payor of last resort only for contract health services (CHS) (See 42 C.F.R. 136.61). In general, Medicaid is considered the payor of last resort.

[35] For more information about private health insurance reform in PPACA, see CRS Report R40942, *Private Health Insurance Provisions in the Patient Protection and Affordable Care Act (PPACA)*, by Hinda Chaikind, Bernadette Fernandez, and Mark Newsom.

[36] See Section 3114 in CRS Report R41 196, *Medicare Provisions in the Patient Protection and Affordable Care Act (PPACA): Summary and Timeline*, coordinated by Patricia A. Davis.

In: Indian Health Care ISBN: 978-1-61942-323-7
Editors J. Hansen and O. Bishop© 2012 Nova Science Publishers, Inc.

Chapter 2

THE INDIAN HEALTH CARE IMPROVEMENT ACT REAUTHORIZATION AND EXTENSION AS ENACTED BY PPACA: DETAILED SUMMARY AND TIMELINE

Elayne J. Heisler

SUMMARY

On March 23, 2010, President Obama signed into law a comprehensive health care reform bill, the Patient Protection and Affordable Care Act (PPACA; P.L. 111-148). Among its provisions, PPACA reenacts, amends, and permanently reauthorizes the Indian Health Care Improvement Act (IHCIA). IHCIA authorizes many specific Indian Health Service (IHS) activities, sets out the national policy for health services administered to Indians, and sets health condition goals for the IHS service population to reduce "the prevalence and incidence of preventable illnesses among, and unnecessary and premature deaths of, Indians." The reauthorization of IHCIA in PPACA amends the IHCIA to, among other changes, expand programs that seek to augment the IHS health care workforce, increase the amount and type of services available at facilities funded by the IHS, and increase the number and type of programs that provide behavioral health and substance abuse treatment to American Indians and Alaska Natives.

This report provides a brief overview of IHCIA and summarizes the provisions of the Indian Health Care Improvement Reauthorization and Extension Act of 2009 as reported by the Senate Committee on Indian Affairs and as enacted and amended by Section 10221 of PPACA. An appendix to this report presents a timeline of the deadlines included in the act.

INTRODUCTION

On March 23, 2010, President Obama signed into law a comprehensive health care reform bill, the Patient Protection and Affordable Care Act (PPACA; P.L. 111-148). Among its provisions, PPACA creates a mandate for most U.S. residents to obtain health insurance and provides for the establishment of insurance exchanges through which certain individuals and families will be able to receive federal subsidies to reduce the cost of purchasing that coverage. The new law expands eligibility for Medicaid; amends the Medicare program in ways that are intended to reduce the growth in Medicare spending that had been projected under preexisting law; imposes an excise tax on insurance plans determined to have high premiums; and makes other changes to the federal tax code, Medicare, Medicaid, and numerous other programs. PPACA also reenacts, amends, and permanently reauthorizes the Indian Health Care Improvement Act (IHCIA).[1] Specifically, Section 10221(a) of PPACA enacted the Indian Health Care Improvement Reauthorization and Extension Act of 2009 (S. 1790),[2] as reported by the Senate Committee on Indian Affairs on December 16, 2009 (hereafter referred to as the IHCIA Reauthorization and Extension Act). Section 10221(b) of PPACA amended sections of the IHCIA Reauthorization and Extension Act (e.g., Sections 111, 134, and 201) and amended one section of IHCIA not included in the IHCIA Reauthorization and Extension Act (Section 806).

IHCIA authorizes many specific IHS activities, sets out the national policy for health services administered to Indians, and sets health condition goals for the IHS service population to reduce "the prevalence and incidence of preventable illnesses among, and unnecessary and premature deaths of, Indians."[3] Prior to PPACA, IHCIA was last fully reauthorized by the Indian Health Amendments of 1992,[4] which extended authorizations of its appropriations through FY2000. The authorizations for all IHCIA programs were later extended through FY200 1.[5] Although authority had expired, IHCIA authorized programs continued to receive annual appropriations since FY2001.

Overview of Indian Health Care

The Indian Health Service (IHS), an agency within the Department of Health and Human Services (HHS), provides health care for approximately 1.9 million eligible American Indians/Alaska Natives through a system of programs and facilities located on or near Indian reservations, and through contractors in certain urban areas.[6] IHS provides services in 35 states, subdivided into 12 geographic "Areas" that consist of one or more states.[7] Each Area is administered by an Area Office; Areas, in turn, are further subdivided into service units that consist of one or more facilities. IHS may provide services directly, or Indian tribes (ITs) or tribal organizations (TOs) may operate IHS facilities and programs themselves through self-determination contracts and self-governance compacts negotiated with IHS.[8] Although most IHS facilities are located on or near reservations, IHS also funds urban Indian health projects (UIHPs), through grants or contracts to urban Indian organizations (UIOs).

The IHCIA authorizes many specific IHS activities, sets out the national policy for health services administered to Indians, and declares that one of the federal goals for the health condition of the IHS service population is to "provide the quantity and quality of health services that will permit the health status of Indians to be raised to the highest possible level.[9] Significantly, IHCIA authorizes direct collections from Medicare, Medicaid, and other third-party insurers. IHCIA also gave IHS authority to grant funding to UIOs, authorizes programs to expand the health care workforce providing services at IHS-funded facilities, and authorized programs that address health concerns for the American Indian and Alaska Native population (e.g., substance abuse, suicide, diabetes).

Overview of Report

This report summarizes the provisions of the IHCIA Reauthorization and Extension Act as enacted by Section 10221 of PPACA. The Act includes two titles. Title I contains amendments to the eight IHCIA titles. Title II amends and reauthorizes the Native Hawaiian Health Care Act,[10] which authorizes health education, health promotion, disease prevention services, and health professions scholarship programs for Native Hawaiians.[11] This report focuses on Title I, which contains eight sections, each of which amends a specific

IHCIA Title. Title I also, with some exceptions, consolidates IHCIA appropriations into a single section, repealing authorizations that had previously been included at the end of each of IHCIA's eight titles. The section numbers below refer to the section numbers in the IHCIA Reauthorization and Extension Act. Where appropriate, sections amended by Section 10221(b) of PPACA are noted. The subtitles below refer to those in the IHCIA Reauthorization and Extension Act, which correspond to the IHCIA title they amend. Each subtitle begins with some background on the IHCIA title it amends to provide context for the descriptions of the law's provisions. **Table 1** describes the major differences between the IHCIA and the IHCIA Reauthorization Extension Act.

Table 1. IHCIA Reauthorization Summary

Title Name and Subject	PPACA
Title I-Indian Health Manpower Authorizes workforce programs to increase the supply of providers at IHS facilities	Maintains title's major sections; repeals section authorizing appropriations for the title; expands use of community health aide workers at IHS-funded facilities; adds a new section funding a demonstration to address IHS health professional shortages; and exempts employees at IHS-funded facilities from certain licensing, registration requirements and related fees.
Title II-Health Services Authorizes IHS health services, research, payments for service-related transportation, payment for services provided through contracts with outside providers (i.e., Contract Health Services (CHS))	Maintains title's major sections; repeals section authorizing appropriations for the title; amends authorization for 2 funds (Indian Health Care Improvement Fund and Catastrophic Health Emergency Fund); expands IHS authority for diabetes, cancer screening, and long-term care programs; and amends sections related to the CHS program.
Title III-Health Facilities Authorizes construction and renovation of IHS facilities; sets procedures by which construction and renovation projects are selected	Maintains title's major sections; repeals section authorizing appropriations for the title; amends IHS construction priority system; and adds new sections requiring grants to build modular and mobile facilities.

Title Name and Subject	PPACA
Title IV-Access to Health Services Authorizes IHS programs to bill Medicare, Medicaid, and private insurance	Maintains title's major sections; repeals section authorizing appropriations for the title; adds the State Children's Health Insurance Program to programs that IHS is authorized to bill; adds new sections permitting ITs, TOs, and UIOS to purchase federal employee health and life insurance benefits for their employees; expands IHS collaboration with the Department of Veterans Affairs and the Department of Defense.
Title V-Health Services for Urban Indians Authorizes grants to UIOs for health projects to serve urban Indians	Maintains title's major sections; repeals section authorizing appropriations for the title; expands grant opportunities available to UIOs.
Title VI-Organization Improvements Establishes IHS's organizational position within HHS; the position of Director of IHS; and requires an automated management information system for IHS record-keeping	Maintains title's major sections; establishes that the IHS Director should report directly to the HHS Secretary; adds new sections requiring: (1) an Office of Direct Service Tribes; and (2) a plan to create a new Nevada Area Office.
Title VII-Behavioral Health Programs Authorizes programs related to behavioral health prevention and treatment	Replaces IHCIA Title VII with new language authorizing new comprehensive behavioral health and treatment programs. Includes a new subsection authorizing programs related to youth suicide prevention.
Title VIII-Miscellaneous Requires the IHS Director to submit a number of reports; establishes IHS eligibility for health services; and defines California Indians, amongst other provisions	Maintains title's major sections; repeals section authorizing appropriations for the title; adds new sections that, among other things, establish: (1) a prescription drugs monitoring program; (2) an IHS Director of HIV/AIDS Prevention and Treatment; and (3) new requirements for the IHS budget requests to reflect inflation and changes in the IHS service population.

Source: CRS analysis of P.L. 94-437, as amended (IHCIA), and P.L. 111-148 (PPACA).

Appendix A includes a detailed timeline of effective dates for the IHCIA Reauthorization and Extension Act provisions. 0 includes a list of acronyms used in this report. The term "Secretary," as used in this report, means the Secretary of HHS, unless otherwise indicated. The term "Indian" in this report refers to "Indian" as defined in IHCIA. Under this definition, an Indian is a person who is a member of a federally recognized tribe, band, nation, or other organized group or community, including any Alaska Native village or group, or regional or village corporation, as defined in or established pursuant to the Alaska Native Claims Settlement Act. [12]

TITLE I—IHCIA REAUTHORIZATION AND AMENDMENTS

Reauthorization, Findings, and Definitions

Sec. 101. Reauthorization

This section amends IHCIA Sec. 825 [25 U.S.C. §1680o] with new language that authorizes an appropriation of such sums as may be necessary to carry out IHCIA for FY20 10 and each fiscal year thereafter to remain available until expended. The section also repeals separate authorizations of appropriations that had been included in each IHCIA title. In addition, it reauthorizes IHCIA indefinitely.

Sec. 102. Findings

This section amends IHCIA Sec. 2 [25 U.S.C. §1601] by adding a new congressional finding that states that providing resources, processes, and structure to eradicate health disparities between Indians and the general population, and that raising Indian health to the highest level are major national goals.

Sec. 103. Declaration of National Indian Health Policy

This section amends IHCIA Sec. 3 [25 U.S.C. §1602] with new language that states that Congress declares that it is the policy of this Nation, in fulfillment of special responsibilities and legal obligations to Indians to (1) ensure the highest possible health status for Indians and urban Indians and to provide all resources necessary to effect that policy; (2) raise Indian and urban Indian health status to that set forth in the Healthy People 2010 or successor objectives; (3) ensure maximum Indian participation in the direction of health care services so as to render the persons administering such services and the services themselves more responsive to the needs and desires of Indian communities; (4) increase the proportion of all degrees in the health professions and allied and associated professions awarded to Indians so that the proportion of Indian health professionals is the same as the general population in each IHS area; (5) require all actions under this Act to be carried out with active and meaningful consultation with ITs and TOs, and conference with UIOs to Indian self-determination; (6) ensure the United States and ITs work in a government-to-government relationship to ensure quality health care for all tribal members; and (7) fund IT and TO-operated programs and facilities at the same level as IHS-operated programs and facilities.

Sec. 104. Definitions

This section amends IHCIA Sec. 4 [25 U.S.C. §1604] by renumbering certain subsections and paragraphs related to specified definitions. The section maintains 12 IHCIA definitions (Area office; fetal alcohol effects; health profession; Indians or Indian; Indian tribe; Secretary; service; service area; substance abuse; urban center; Urban Indian; Urban Indian Organization), amends definitions for 5 terms (disease prevention, fetal alcohol syndrome (FAS), health promotion, service unit, and tribal organization) and adds 12 new terms, for a total of 29 terms. The 12 new terms are "behavioral health," "California Indians," "community college," "contract health service," "Department," "Indian Health Program," "junior or community college," "reservation," "telehealth," "telemedicine," "tribal college or university," and "Tribal Health Program."

This report uses the following terms, as they are used in the IHCIA Reauthorization and Extension Act, to refer to different types of Indian facilities that are eligible for a given program: "Indian Health Program" (IHP), which is defined as any health program administered by the IHS or by an IT or TO under either the Indian Self-Determination and Education Assistance Act, as amended (ISDEAA),[13] or the Buy Indian Act;[14] and "Tribal Health Program" (THP), which is defined as any IT or TO operating a health program under ISDEAA. THPs are included within the term IHP.

Subtitle A—Indian Health Manpower[15]

Subtitle A includes sections that amend IHCIA Title I "Indian Health Manpower." This title includes provisions related to personnel recruitment, scholarships, and other educational programs that seek to augment the Indian health workforce. IHS has high vacancy rates in many of its health professions—25% for physicians, 15% for dentists, and 16% for nurses, for instance, as of December 2009.[16] These vacancy rates are higher than those of federally funded health centers in rural areas, facilities that also have a difficult time recruiting providers.[17] The purpose of IHCIA Title I is to increase the number, and also enhance the skills, of Indian and non-Indian health professionals and other health personnel in the IHS.

PPACA maintains a number of existing sections that authorize scholarships for preparatory and professional schools. It also authorizes new programs that may expand the workforce at IHS, IT, TO, and UIO facilities. Specifically, it authorizes programs that may expand the use of community health workers outside of Alaska, may increase the number of providers at facilities with severe shortages, and it amends licensing requirements for UIO providers to facilitate UIOs provider recruitment.

Sec. 111. Community Health Aide Program[18]

This section amends IHCIA Sec. 119 [25 U.S.C. §1616l] with new language that requires the Secretary, under authority of the Snyder Act, to develop and operate a Community Health Aide Program (CHAP) in Alaska, under which IHS is to train Alaska Natives to provide health care, health promotion, and disease prevention in rural Alaska Native villages. The section requires the Secretary to provide, in a specified manner, a high standard of training to community health aides; establish teleconferencing capacity in health clinics located in or near those villages for use of CHAPs or community health practitioners; establish and maintain a CHAP certification board; and provide continuing education, close supervision, and a system to review and evaluate CHAP work. The section also prohibits a CHAP dental health aide therapist from performing certain pulpal therapy or extractions without a determination of a medical emergency by a licensed dentist and from performing any other oral or jaw surgeries except for uncomplicated extractions.

The section requires the Secretary, acting through IHS, to establish a neutral review panel to study the CHAP dental health aide therapist program to ensure that the quality of care is adequate and appropriate. The section specifies panel membership, the factors of the study, and requires consultation with Alaska tribal organizations, and a report to Congress.

The section also authorizes the expansion of CHAP, except for the dental health aide therapist program, into a national program, but requires that the expansion not reduce Alaska CHAP funding. The section exempts ITs and TOs using dental health aides from certain specified instructional requirements for ITs or TOs located in states (other than Alaska) that permit, under state law, dental health aide therapists or midlevel health providers to supply such services. The section requires the Secretary, acting through the IHS, to facilitate the implementation of dental health aide programs by ITs and TOs who elect to provide these services; and prohibits the Secretary from filling IHS program vacancies for certified dentists with dental health aides. The section further specifies that nothing in this section restricts the ability of IHS, an IT, or a TO to participate in any program or to provide any service authorized in any other federal law.

Sec. 112. Health Professional Chronic Shortage Demonstration Programs

This section adds a new IHCIA Sec. 123 *Health Professional Chronic Shortage Demonstration Programs* [25 U.S.C. §1616p], which authorizes the Secretary, acting through IHS, to fund demonstration programs for IHPs to address chronic shortages of health professionals. The section specifies the purposes of the demonstration programs, and requires that the program incorporate an advisory board composed of representatives from tribes, IHPs, and Indian communities served by the program.

Sec. 113. Exemption from Payment of Certain Fees

This section adds a new IHCIA Sec. 124 *Exemption of Payment of Certain Fees* [25 U.S.C. §1616q], which exempts employees of a THP or UIO from the payment of licensing, registration, and other fees imposed by a federal agency, to the same extent that Public Health Service (PHS) Commissioned Corps officers or other IHS employees are exempt from the fees.

Subtitle B — Health Services

Subtitle B includes sections that amend IHCIA Title II "Health Services" authorizing a number of specific non-behavioral health programs and activities, including prevention activities, diabetes and cancer programs, Indian men's health, Indian school health education programs, research and epidemiological centers, and a fund for the elimination of funding inequities among health care programs. PPACA amends a number of programs in this title. It also authorizes a report that studies and makes recommendations about contract health service (CHS) funding and how IHS funding is distributed across IHS service areas. CHS refers to services that IHS, ITs, or TOs may purchase, through contract, from private providers in instances where the THP cannot provide the needed care.

Sec. 121. Indian Health Care Improvement Fund

This section amends IHCIA Sec. 201 [25 U.S.C. §1621] with new language that authorizes the Secretary, acting through IHS, to use funds designated as the "Indian Health Care Improvement Fund" (IHCIF), to eliminate tribes' deficiencies in health status and resources (as defined in the section), eliminate backlogs in provision of health care to Indians, meet health needs efficiently and equitably, eliminate inequities in funding for both direct care and CHS, and augment the ability of IHS to meet 10 specified health service responsibilities. The Secretary is authorized to expend IHCIF funds either directly or through contracts or compacts under ISDEAA. The section also prohibits using funds appropriated under this section to offset funds appropriated under other laws, permits IHCIF allocation among service units and THPs, and requires the Secretary to determine (in consultation with the affected ITs and TOs) the apportionment of funds among service units, ITs, and TOs for the specified health service responsibilities. The section also requires that THPs be equally eligible for funds with IHS programs and requires that appropriations under this section be included in the base budget of the IHS for subsequent fiscal years. The section requires the Secretary to submit a report to Congress three years after enactment on the current health status and resource deficiencies for each tribe or service unit, and specifies the data to be included in this report. In addition, the section specifies that nothing in the section is intended to diminish the primary responsibility of the IHS to eliminate backlogs in unmet health care or to discourage additional efforts by IHS to achieve parity among tribes.

Sec. 122. Catastrophic Health Emergency Fund

This section replaces IHCIA Sec. 202 [25 U.S.C. §1621a] with new language that establishes the Catastrophic Health Emergency Fund (CHEF), administered by the Secretary through IHS headquarters, to meet extraordinary medical costs associated with the treatment of victims of disasters or catastrophic illnesses. The section specifies the uses, administration, and regulations of this fund. It also specifies that CHEF consists of appropriations and third-party reimbursements to which IHS is entitled for treatments paid for by CHEF, and requires that no part of the CHEF or the administration thereof be subject to contract or grant (including those made under ISDEAA). It prohibits CHEF from being apportioned on an Area Office, Service Unit, or any other basis. The section also prohibits funds appropriated to CHEF from being used to offset or limit other IHS appropriations and it requires that all reimbursements to which IHS is entitled from any source, by reason of treatment rendered to any victim of a disaster or catastrophic illness, the cost of which was paid from CHEF, be deposited into CHEF.

Sec. 123. Diabetes Prevention, Treatment, and Control

This section inserts a new IHCIA Sec. 204 *Diabetes Prevention, Treatment, and Control* [25 U.S.C. §1621c], which requires the Secretary, acting through IHS and in consultation with ITs and TOs, to determine the incidence of diabetes and its complications among Indians and, based on the incidence determined, what actions IHS service units need to take to prevent, treat, and control the disease, including effective ongoing monitoring. The Secretary is required—to the extent indicated and with medical consent—to screen Indians for diabetes and for conditions that indicate a high risk for diabetes. The section also permits screening through Internet-based programs, and requires the Secretary to establish a cost-effective approach to ensure ongoing monitoring of diabetes indicators. In addition, the Secretary is required to maintain model diabetes projects in existence at enactment, and is required to provide recurring funding to ITs and THPs for diabetes projects that these entities operate under this section, including funding for projects in existence at enactment and funded thereafter.

In addition, the section authorizes the Secretary to provide dialysis programs for IHS, ITs, and TOs, including equipment and staffing. The Secretary is also required to consult with the ITs and TOs in each IHS area on diabetes programs, establish diabetes patient registries in each IHS Area Office, and ensure that the data collected are disseminated to other Area Offices. The section also authorizes diabetes control officers in each IHS Area Office and states that any activity carried out by a diabetes control officer that is the subject of a contract or compact of ISDEAA , and any funds made available to carry out these activities may not be divisible for the purposes of ISDEAA.

Sec. 124. Other Authority for Provision of Services and Long-Term Care

This section inserts a new IHCIA Sec. 205 [25 U.S.C. §1621d], which authorizes the Secretary to provide funding, through programs and services of

IHS, ITs, and TOs, for health-care-related services and programs (not otherwise specified in IHCIA) for hospice care, assisted living, longterm care, and home- and community-based services (as defined in this section). The section also specifies eligibility criteria for long-term care services, authorizes funding through IHS, ITs, and TOs, for "convenient care services" pursuant to IHCIA Sec. 307(c)(2)(A), and repeals IHCIA Sec. 821, which had authorized a demonstration for home-and community based services.

This section also amends IHCIA Sec. 822 [25 U.S.C. §1680l] by authorizing the Secretary, acting through the IHS, to provide, directly or through ISDEAA contracts or compacts with THPs, longterm care and health care services associated with long-term care at any long-term care or related facility owned or operated by a THP directly or under ISDEAA. The section requires that the agreements provide for sharing staff and other services between an IHS facility and the contracting IT's or TO's facility. The section authorizes such contracts to allow delegation to the contractors of necessary supervision over IHS employees, and permits ITs and TOs to construct, renovate, or expand nursing facilities. The section also specifies certain terms of the agreement, including funding allocations, and specifies that any nursing facility funded under this section must meet the requirements for such facilities under Medicare statute. The section requires the Secretary to provide necessary technical and other assistance to tribal applicants, and encourages the use of existing underused facilities and permits the use of swing beds, for long-term or similar care.

Sec. 125 Third Parties Reimbursements

This section amends IHCIA Sec. 206 [25 U.S.C. §1621e] by inserting new language that permits the United States, ITs, and TOs the right to recover reasonable charges billed (or, if higher, the highest amount a third party would pay for care and services from a non-governmental provider) for health services provided by these entities to an individual, to the same extent that the individual or any nongovernmental provider of health services would be eligible to receive reimbursement or indemnification. The section specifies that entities from whom recovery can occur include insurance companies, health maintenance organizations, employee benefit plans, third-party tortfeasors, state political subdivisions, local governments, or any other responsible or liable third parties. The section limits the right of recovery against any state to circumstances where the health services are covered under workers' compensation laws or a no-fault automobile accident insurance plan. The section prohibits state or local laws, contract provisions, insurance or health maintenance organization policies, employee benefit plans, self-insurance plans, managed care plans, or other health care plans or programs entered into or renewed after November 23, 1988, from preventing or hindering the right of recovery. The section also prohibits any action by the United States, an IT, or a TO from affecting the right of an injured person to collect for the portion of their damages not covered hereunder. In addition, the section permits the United States, an IT, or a TO to enforce the right of recovery by intervening or joining in specified civil actions or proceedings, or by instituting a separate civil action (after notifying the individual or his representatives or heirs), and requires reasonable efforts to notify the individual. The section also authorizes ITs or TOs, independent of the rights of the injured or diseased person, to recover from tortfeasors or their insurers the reasonable value of health services provided or paid in accordance with the Federal Medical Care Recovery Act.

The section prohibits the U.S. from recovering from an IT's, TO's, or UIO's self-insurance plan, but allows recovery from a tribe if the tribal governing body provides specific written authorization for a specified time period and permits expenditure of amounts recovered to provide additional health services. The section requires the awarding of reasonable attorneys fees and costs of litigation to prevailing plaintiffs under this section, prohibits specified health insurance and related entities from denying reimbursement of an IHS or IT's or TO's claim on the basis of the claim's format (if the format meets certain standards), and applies a specified statute of limitations.[19] The section applies to UIOs the same rights of recovery, for the populations they serve, as those allowed to ITs and TOs for their served populations. The section also provides that nothing in it limits the right of the United States, an IT, or a TO to recover under any applicable federal, state, or tribal law, including medical lien laws.

Sec. 126. Crediting of Reimbursements

This section amends IHCIA Sec. 207 [25 U.S.C. §1621f] with language that requires that— except as provided under IHCIA Sec. 202 regarding the CHEF or under IHCIA Sec. 813 regarding services to ineligible persons—all reimbursements received or recovered for provision of health service by IHS, an IT, a TO, or a UIO are required to be credited to the respective entity (including the service unit providing the health service). The section requires that reimbursements be used as specified under IHCIA Sec. 401 ("Sec. 151. Treatment of Payments under SSA Health Benefits Programs"). The section also prohibits IHS from offsetting or limiting the amounts obligated to any service unit, or any entity receiving IHS funding, because of the receipt of reimbursements under this section.

Sec. 127. Behavioral Health Training and Community Education Programs

This section amends IHCIA Sec. 209 [25 U.S.C. §1621h] by inserting new language requiring the HHS Secretary, acting through IHS, and the Secretary of the Interior, in consultation with IT and TOs, to conduct a study and compile a list of specified types of staff positions within the Bureau of Indian Affairs (BIA), IHS, ITs, and TOs, whose qualifications should include training in the identification, prevention, education, referral, or treatment of mental illness, dysfunction, or self-destructive behavior. The appropriate secretary is required to provide culturally relevant training criteria appropriate for each type of position and to ensure that this training has been or will be provided. IHS is also required, upon request by a IT, TO, or UIO, to develop and implement a program of community education on mental illness, or assist the requester with doing so. The section specifies that when the positions are funded under ISDEAA the appropriate secretary is required to ensure that training costs are included in the contract or compact. The section also requires the IHS to provide technical assistance for obtaining and developing community education materials. Within 90 days of enactment, the HHS Secretary is required to develop a plan, to be implemented under the Snyder Act, to increase behavioral health services by at least 500 staff positions within five years, with at least 200 of such positions devoted to child, adolescent, and family services.

Sec. 128. Cancer Screening

This section amends IHCIA Sec. 212 [25 U.S.C. §1621k] by adding that mammography be provided under standards established by the Secretary under the SSA, to ensure the safety and accuracy of the mammography and other cancer screenings.

Sec. 129. Patient Travel Costs

This section amends IHCIA Sec. 213 [25 U.S.C. §1621l] to insert new language that authorizes the Secretary, through IHS, to provide funds for specified patient travel costs associated with receiving IHS-funded health care services (those provided directly by IHS or through ISDEAA contract or compact). These services include emergency air transport and non-emergency air transport where ground transport is not feasible; transportation by ambulance, specially equipped vehicle, or private vehicle where no other transportation is available; or other means required when air or motor vehicle transport is not available. The section also authorizes the Secretary to provide funding for qualified escorts, as defined in the section.

Sec. 130. Epidemiology Centers

This section amends IHCIA Sec. 214 [25 U.S.C. §1621m] with new language that requires the Secretary to establish an epidemiology center in each IHS Area to carry out seven specified functions, in consultation with ITs, TOs, or UIOs. The section specifies that an epidemiology center is subject to ISDEAA. The section also requires that the Director of the Centers for Disease Control and Prevention (CDC) provide technical assistance to these epidemiology centers. The section also authorizes the Secretary to make grants to ITs, TOs, and UIOs, and eligible intertribal consortia (as defined) to operate an epidemiology center and to conduct epidemiological studies of Indian communities, and specifies the criteria for applicants and the uses of such grants. The section further requires that epidemiology centers operated under such grants be treated as public health authorities for purposes of the Health Insurance Portability and Accountability Act[20] (HIPAA). In addition, the section requires the Secretary to grant such centers access to and use of data, data sets, monitoring systems, delivery systems, and other protected health information in the Secretary's possession, and specifies that such centers' activities are, for purposes of HIPAA, for research or disease prevention and control.

Sec. 131. Indian Youth Grant Program

This section amends IHCIA Sec. 216(b)(2) [25 U.S.C. §1621o] by striking reference to Section 209(m) regarding prohibited uses of grant funds and inserts reference to Section 708(c), regarding intermediate adolescent behavioral health services ("Sec. 708. Indian Youth Program").

Sec. 132. American Indians into Psychology program

This section amends IHCIA Sec. 217 [25 U.S.C. §1621p] by replacing it with new language that authorizes the Secretary, acting through the IHS director, to establish a grant program to award grants of not more than $300,000 to nine colleges and universities for developing and maintaining Indian psychology career recruitment programs. The section requires that one grant be awarded to the University of North Dakota to establish a Quentin N. Burdick American Indians into Psychology Program. The section also requires that grants be awarded to locations throughout the United States to maximize their availability to Indian students, including awarding grants to locations that had not previously operated programs. In addition, the section requires the Secretary to issue regulations for competitive funding, and specifies conditions of the grants, including recipients' service obligations. The section authorizes to be appropriated $2.7 million for FY20 10 and for each fiscal year thereafter.

Sec. 133. Projects Related to Communicable and Infectious Diseases

This section strikes IHCIA Sec. 218 [25 U.S.C. §1621q] replacing it with new language that authorizes the Secretary to make grants to ITs and TOs for projects to prevent, control, and eliminate communicable and infectious diseases, provide public information and education on such diseases, provide education and skills improvement activities on such diseases for health professionals, and establish demonstration projects for the screening, treatment, and prevention of the hepatitis C virus. Grant recipients are encouraged to coordinate their activities with the CDC and state and local health agencies. The section also authorizes the Secretary to provide technical assistance, upon request, and requires the Secretary to make a biennial report to Congress.

Sec. 134. Licensing[21]

This section amends IHCIA Sec. 221 [25 U.S.C. §1621t] to exempt licensed health care professionals from state licensing requirements while employed by a THP providing services under an ISDEAA contract or compact.

This section also amends IHCIA Sec. 106 [25 U.S.C. §1615] to insert new language that authorizes the Secretary to provide programs or allowances to encourage specified health professionals and scholarship and stipend recipients under IHCIA Sections 104 (Indian health professions scholarships), 105 (IHS extern programs), 106 (Community Education Allowances), and 115 (Health Training Programs for Community Colleges) to join or continue in an IHP, and to work in rural or remote areas where significant numbers of Indians reside. These programs or allowances include licensing and board or certification examination assistance that may be used to help individuals to transition into IHPs. The section also authorizes the Secretary to provide technical assistance to these health professionals to assist them with fulfilling their service obligations. The section also authorizes programs and allowances for IHS and tribal health professionals to take leave of their duty stations for a period of time each year for specified continuing professional education.

Sec. 135. Liability for Payment

This section amends IHCIA Sec. 222 [25 U.S.C. §1621u] to exempt a patient who receives HIS-authorized CHS from being held liable for any charges or costs associated with those authorized services. The section also requires the Secretary to notify, within five business days of the provider receiving a claim, the CHS provider and the patient who receives the services that the patient is not liable for the claim. The section prohibits the CHS provider from recourse against the patient for payment if the notice has been received or if the claim has been deemed accepted under IHCIA Sec. 220(b) (CHS claims that IHS failed to respond to in the allotted time).

Sec. 136. Offices of Indian Men's Health and Indian Women's Health

This section amends IHCIA Sec. 223 [25 U.S.C. §1621v] to insert new language that authorizes the Secretary, acting through IHS, to establish an office within IHS known as the "Office of Indian Men's Health." The section specifies that a director heads the office and coordinates and promotes the health status of Indian men in the United States. The section requires that the Secretary, acting through IHS, submit a report to Congress describing the activities carried out by the director and any findings with respect to the health of Indian men. The section also requires the Secretary, acting through IHS, to establish an "Office of Indian Women's Health" to monitor and improve the quality of Indian women's health of all ages.

Sec. 137. CHS Administration and Disbursement Formula

This section adds a new IHCIA Sec. 226 *Contract Health Service Administration and Disbursement Formula* [25 U.S.C. §1621y], which requires the Government Accountability Office (GAO) to submit a report, as soon as practicable after enactment, to specified congressional committees and the Secretary, and make it available to each IT, regarding specified elements of the CHS program. Upon receipt of the report, the Secretary is required to consult with ITs regarding the program, including its funding distribution, to determine the adequacy of the current funding formula, and any modifications that are required for the program to be funded at such level as GAO may recommend. The Secretary is authorized, following this consultation, to initiate procedures to negotiate or promulgate regulations to establish a disbursement formula for future CHS program funding.

Subtitle C — Health Facilities

Subtitle C includes sections that amend IHCIA Title III "Health Facilities." This title includes sections related to health care and sanitation facilities. IHS funds the construction, equipping, and maintenance of hospitals, health centers, clinics, and other health care delivery facilities operated by IHS and tribes. IHS also funds the construction of water supply and sewage facilities and solid waste disposal systems, and provides technical assistance for the operation and maintenance of such facilities.

PPACA sets new requirements for the priority system for building and renovating facilities and new requirements for closure of IHS-operated health care facilities. It also authorizes demonstration projects to increase the number of facilities available to provide services to American Indians and Alaska Natives including demonstration projects for funding mobile and modular health facilities–two mechanisms considered to build health facilities more rapidly. As discussed below, IHS maintains a priority system to determine which facilities will be built and in what order. The agency also notes that due to funding constraints some facility construction or renovation projects are completed in phases, which may delay completion and increase costs.[22]

Sec. 141. Health Care Facilities Priority System

This section amends IHCIA Sec. 301 [25 U.S.C. §1631] to require the Secretary, acting through IHS, to maintain a health care facility priority system developed in consultation with ITs and TOs that prioritizes tribal needs, includes the methodology for prioritization, and allows for the nomination of new projects at least once every three years. The priority list may also include the top 10 priority facilities for four specified types of facilities as well as other facilities or needs that IHS may identify. The section requires that the Secretary ensure that the planning, design, construction, renovation, and expansion of facilities operated under ISDEAA are fully and equitably integrated into the health care facility priority system. The section also prohibits a project's priority in effect at enactment from being affected by a new facility priority system if the project meets specified criteria and was identified in the FY2008 IHS budget justification as being in the top 10 for four specified types of facilities.[23]

The section also defines the Facilities Appropriations Advisory Board and a Facilities Needs Assessment Workgroup,[24] and requires—not later than one year after enactment—the Secretary to submit to specified committees of Congress an initial report with a national ranked list of all IHS, IT, and TO health care facilities needs developed for the board and workgroup, and requires the Secretary to update the report every five years beginning in 2011. The section also requires the Secretary to submit to the President, for inclusion in reports to Congress,[25] an annual report describing the new health care facility priority system and its methodology, and listing top 10 facilities for four specified types of facilities with justifications and projected costs. The Secretary is required to prepare this annual report in consultation with ITs, TOs, and UIOs and is required to review the ITs' and TOs' total unmet facility needs. The section also requires the GAO to study the methodologies used by IHS in developing the health care facility priority system and in making facility needs assessments, and to report to specified committees of Congress and the Secretary. The section further requires the Secretary to consult with ITs and TOs, and confer with UIOs in developing innovative approaches to address unmet facility needs; and makes facility funds appropriated under the Snyder Act subject to ISDEAA.

Sec. 142. Priority of Certain Projects Protected

This section amends IHCIA Sec. 301 [25 U.S.C. §1631] to add a new subsection that prohibits a project's priority in effect at enactment from being affected by a new facility priority system (see "Sec. 141. Health Care Facilities Priority System" above) if the project was identified in the FY2008 IHS budget justification as being in the top 10 for the four specified types of facilities; had completed both Phase I and Phase II of the construction priority system in effect prior to enactment; or is selected by the Secretary on the Secretary's initiative or pursuant to an IT or TO request.

Sec. 143. Indian Health Care Delivery Demonstration Project

This section amends IHCIA Sec. 307 [25 U.S.C. §1637] by inserting new language that authorizes the Secretary to make grants to, or construction contracts or agreements with, ITs and TOs under ISDEAA to establish demonstration projects to test alternative health care delivery systems through health facilities to Indians, including through construction and renovation of hospitals, health centers, health stations, and other facilities or through cooperative agreements or other arrangements with other health care providers. The section specifies the uses of funds and permits their use to match federal and other funds. The section requires that equal criteria be used in evaluating tribal and IHS facilities, and requires integration of ISDEAA facility planning and construction into demonstration projects. The section defines "convenient care services" as any primary care service that is offered in an alternative setting or outside of regular working hours. The section also authorizes the Secretary to permit demonstration projects meeting certain specified criteria and gives preference to demonstration projects that meet these criteria and are located in the following Service Units: Cass Lake, MN; Mescaleroa, NM; Owyhee and Elko, NV; Schurz, NV; and Ft. Yuma, CA.

In addition, the section requires the Secretary to promulgate regulations for application approval; it also establishes granting criteria, the grant selection process, and the requirements for technical assistance. The section also permits facilities, under the demonstration projects, to provide services to otherwise ineligible persons—that is, those who are not eligible for IHS services—and extends hospital privileges in IHS facilities to non-IHS health practitioners.

Sec. 144. Tribal Management of Federally Owned Quarters

This section adds a new IHCIA Sec. 309 *Tribal Management of Federally Owned Quarters* [25 U.S.C. § 1 638a], which authorizes THPs operating a health care facility and the associated federally owned quarters pursuant to an ISDEAA contract or compact to establish reasonable rental rates for the federally owned quarters, by notifying the Secretary, and to collect the rent directly. The section sets the objectives of the THP 's rental rates, requires that such quarters remain eligible for improvement and repair funds to the same extent as federally owned quarters, and requires at least 60-days notice before changes in the rental rate. In addition, the section specifies requirements for direct rent collection by a THP, requires federal employees subject to the rent to pay the THP directly, and sets the effective date for a retrocession of rent collection authority. The provision also permits rental rates in Alaska to be comparable to those in the nearest established community with a year-round population of 1,500.

Sec. 145. Other Funding for Facilities

This section adds a new IHCIA Sec. 311 *Other Funding, Equipment, and Supplies for Facilities* [25 U.S.C. §1638e], which authorizes the head of any federal agency that funds equipment or other supplies used for the planning, design, construction, or operation or a health care or sanitation facility (as defined) to transfer funds, equipment, or supplies to the Secretary. These transfers must be used for the planning, design, or construction of a health care or sanitation facility in accordance with the IHCIA, and with the purposes for which the funds were made available to the transferring agency. The section also authorizes the Secretary to accept such funds and use equipment and supplies for the planning, design, construction, and operation of health care and sanitation facilities for Indians, including facilities operated under ISDEAA contracts or compacts. In addition, the section states that funds received under this section must not affect facility priority established under IHCIA Sec. 301.

The section also authorizes the Secretary to enter into interagency agreements with federal or state agencies or other entities to accept funds, equipments, or supplies to plan, design, construct health care or sanitation facilities to be administered by an IHP in order to carry out the purposes of IHCIA or the purposes for which the funds were appropriated or provided. The section requires the Secretary, acting through IHS, to establish, by regulation, standards for the planning design, construction, and operation of health care or sanitation facilities serving Indians under IHCIA; and requires that, notwithstanding other provisions of law, other applicable HHS regulations apply to funds transferred under this section.

Sec. 146. Modular Component Facilities Demonstration Program

This section adds a new IHCIA Sec. 312 *Indian Country Modular Component Facilities Demonstration Program* [25 U.S.C. §1638f], which requires the Secretary, acting through the IHS, to establish a demonstration program to award grants for the establishment of not less than three modular component health care facilities (as defined). Grants will be awarded for the purchase, installation, and maintenance of such facilities in Indian communities for the provision of health care services. The section requires the Secretary to solicit petitions from ITs for modular component health care facilities; establishes petition criteria; and specifies that the Secretary is required to give priority to projects already on the IHS facilities construction priority list and to applications that demonstrate that modular facilities can be constructed more quickly and more economically than traditional facilities while adequately meeting health care service needs. The section also specifies that entities receiving grants under this section are not eligible for entry on the facilities construction priority list in FY2011 or any successor lists. ITs are eligible for grants under this section regardless of their participation in ISDEAA contracts or compacts. ITs and TOs receiving funds under this section are subject to ISDEAA. This section also requires the Secretary to submit a report, not later than one year after grants are awarded, describing grant activities and potential benefits. Finally, the section authorizes $50 million to be appropriated for the first five fiscal years and such sums as may be necessary in subsequent fiscal years.

Sec. 147. Mobile Health Stations Demonstration Program

This section adds a new IHCIA Sec. 313 *Mobile Health Demonstration Program* [25 U.S.C. §1638g], which requires the Secretary, acting through the IHS, to establish a demonstration project to award funds for uses specified, including providing specialty health care (as defined) to at least three mobile health station projects (as defined by this section). Tribal consortia (as defined) are eligible for grants under this section after submitting a petition to the Secretary with required information. The Secretary is also required to submit a report to Congress, not later than one year after the demonstration has been established, describing and evaluating the demonstration program's activities and benefits. There are authorized to be appropriated $5 million for each of the first five fiscal years and such sums as may be necessary for each fiscal year thereafter to carry out the grant program under this section.

Subtitle D — Access to Health Services

Subtitle D amends IHCIA's Title IV "Access to Health Services," which authorizes IHS health care facilities to receive reimbursements from SSA's Medicare and Medicaid programs. This authorization was a major component of the original IHCIA passed in 1976. The title establishes a "special fund" to receive the reimbursements and specifies what they can be used for. These reimbursements are an important source of funds for IHS. In FY20 10, IHS estimated that it received about $735 million from reimbursements.[26] These reimbursements are used to augment services received at IHS-funded facilities because IHCIA excludes Medicare or Medicaid reimbursements from being considered when determining annual Indian health appropriations. Other non-IHCIA sections of PPACA also make changes to IHS-funded facilities' ability to bill SSA programs and include provisions to increase American Indian and Alaska Native enrollment in these programs.

PPACA adds the State Children's Health Insurance Program (CHIP) to the programs that IHS health care facilities may bill, and expands the ability of THPs to bill these programs directly. In addition to amendments related to SSA programs, this subtitle also includes sections related to private insurance and sections related to coordination between IHS, the Department of Veterans Affairs (VA), and the Department of Defense (DOD).

Sec. 151. Treatment of Payments under SSA Health Benefits Programs

This section amends IHCIA Sec. 401 [25 U.S.C. §1641] to require that payments received by an IHP or a UIO from Medicare, Medicaid, or CHIP may not be considered in determining appropriations for Indian health care services. The section prohibits the Secretary from providing services to Indians with coverage under Medicare, Medicaid, or CHIP in preference to those Indians without such coverage. The section also requires that Medicare and Medicaid payments to IHS facilities be placed in a special fund held by the Secretary, and requires the Secretary to ensure that each IHS service unit receives 100% of the reimbursed amounts to which the service unit's facilities are entitled.

The section requires that amounts in the special fund be used by a facility first (to the extent provided in appropriations acts) to improve IHS facilities so they can comply with the applicable conditions and requirements of Medicare or Medicaid; if the reimbursed amounts are in excess of the amount necessary to make such improvements, the facilities are required to use the funds— after consulting with the tribes being served by the service unit—to reduce health resource deficiencies of Indian tribes, including for additional services authorized in IHCIA Sec. 205 ("Sec. 124. Other Authority for Provision of Services and Long-Term Care").

In addition, the section excludes THPs electing to receive payments directly from Medicare or Medicaid—called direct billing—from making payments into, or receiving from, the special fund. The section authorizes a THP to elect to directly bill and receive payments from Medicare, Medicaid, CHIP, or other third-party payors. The section requires that payments be used to improve THP facilities so they can comply with the applicable conditions and requirements of Medicare, Medicaid, or CHIP; or that payments be used to provide additional health care services, or to otherwise achieve the objectives in IHCIA Sec. 3 ("Sec. 103. Declaration of National Indian Health Policy"). The section also subjects THP direct payments to all auditing requirements applicable to whichever programs it chooses to bill directly and to all auditing requirements applicable to the IHP. The section requires that a THP receiving reimbursements or payments under Medicare, Medicaid, or CHIP provide to IHS a list of each provider enrollment number (or other identifier) under which the THP receives such reimbursements or payments and requires that IHS share this and other necessary information with the Centers for Medicare and Medicaid Services (CMS), the agency that administers the Medicare, Medicaid, and CHIP programs. The section also requires the Secretary, with assistance from CMS, to examine and implement any administrative changes that facilitate direct billing and reimbursement, including agreements with states necessary to provide for direct billing under Medicaid or CHIP. The section also permits participants (i.e., THPs) to withdraw from the program under the same conditions that an IT or TO may retrocede a contracted program under ISDEAA. In addition, the section authorizes the Secretary to terminate a direct billing participant if the Secretary determines that the participant has failed to comply with certain specified requirements, but requires the Secretary to provide notice and an opportunity to correct the noncompliance. The section cross-references specified sections of the SSA relating to the special fund and the direct billing program.

Sec. 152. Purchasing Health Care Coverage

This section amends IHCIA Sec. 402 [25 U.S.C. §1642] to authorize ITs, TOs, or UIOs to use funds made available for health benefits for IHS beneficiaries under SSA programs, the ISDEAA (except for funds under IHCIA Sec. 402), or other law (except for Sec. 404) to purchase health benefits coverage. This may include coverage for service within a contract health service delivery area (CHSDA)[27] or any portion of a CHSDA that would have otherwise been provided by CHS; coverage through a tribally owned and operated health care plan, a state or locally authorized or licensed health care plan, a health insurance provider or managed care organization, or a self- insured plan. The section permits that purchased coverage be based on the financial needs of the individual beneficiaries (as determined by the tribe(s) being served) and permits funds to be used to operate a self-insured plan.

Sec. 153. SSA Health Benefit Programs Outreach and Enrollment Grants

This section amends IHCIA Sec. 404 [25 U.S.C. §1644] to require the Secretary to make grants or enter into contracts with ITs and TOs for programs on or near reservations, trust lands, including using electronics and telecommunications, to assist individual Indians to enroll in Medicare, Medicaid, and CHIP, and other health benefit programs, and pay premiums and cost sharing required by the programs.[28] Payment of premiums and cost sharing may be based on need as determined by the IT or TO. The section also requires the Secretary, acting through IHS, to place conditions as deemed necessary on the contracts and grants, including requirements to determine Indian Medicaid, Medicare, and CHIP populations, educate Indians about the programs' benefits, provide transportation, and develop and implement methods to improve Indian participation in the programs. The section also applies the enrollment, premium, and cost- sharing assistance program to UIOs for the populations they serve, and sets requirements for agreements with such organizations. The section also requires the Secretary, acting through CMS, to consult with states, IHS, ITs, TOs, and UIOs on developing and disseminating best practices to facilitate agreements between the states, ITs, TOs, and UIOs regarding enrollment and retention of Indians in Medicare, Medicaid, and CHIP. The section cross references SSA Sec. 1139 regarding agreements for collecting, preparing, and submitting applications for Medicaid and CHIP. The section also defines the terms "premium" and "cost sharing."

Sec. 154. Sharing Arrangements with Federal Agencies

This section amends IHCIA Sec. 405 [25 U.S.C. §1645] to insert new language that authorizes the Secretary to enter into or expand arrangements for IHS, ITs, and TOs to share medical facilities and services with the VA and the DOD, but requires consultation with affected tribes prior to finalizing an arrangement. The section prohibits the Secretary from taking any action under this section that impairs (1) an Indian's priority access to, or eligibility for, health care services provided through IHS; (2) a veteran's priority access to VA health care services; (3) the quality of IHS health care provided to an Indian; (4) the quality of VA or DOD health care; or (5) an Indian veteran's eligibility to receive VA health care. The section requires reimbursement to the IHS, ITs, or TOs by the VA or DOD where beneficiaries eligible for VA or DOD services receive care from the IHS, ITs, or TOs. The section prohibits construing the section as creating any right of a non-Indian veteran to IHS health services.

Sec. 155. Eligible Indian Veteran Services

This section adds a new IHCIA Sec. 407 *Eligible Indian Veteran Services* [25 U.S.C. §1647], which makes a congressional finding that collaborations between the Secretary and the VA for treatment of Indian veterans at IHS facilities and increased enrollment for VA services by Indian tribal veterans should both be encouraged to the maximum extent practicable. The section also reaffirms the goals of a 2003 memorandum of understanding between IHS and VA's Veterans Health Administration regarding VA-authorized treatment of eligible Indian veterans at IHS facilities. The section requires the Secretary to provide for payment for veteran-related, VA- authorized treatment under a local memorandum of understanding. The section requires the Secretary to establish guidelines for such payments to the VA, and prohibits use of funds appropriated for IHS facilities, CHS, or contract support costs to make such payments. The section also requires the Secretary to consult with affected tribes in negotiating local memoranda of understanding, and defines "eligible Indian veteran" and "local memorandum of understanding."

Sec. 156. Nondiscrimination Under Federal Health Care Programs

This section adds a new IHCIA Sec. 408 *Nondiscrimination Under Federal Health Care Programs in Qualifications for Reimbursement for Services* [25 U.S.C. §1647a], which requires federal health care programs to accept an entity operated by IHS, an IT, TO, or a UIO, as a provider eligible to receive payment for health care services furnished to an Indian on the same basis as other qualified providers, if the Indian entity meets generally applicable state or other requirements for providers. The section requires that any requirement that providers be licensed or recognized under state or local law be deemed to have been met by such an Indian entity if the entity meets all applicable standards for licensure, regardless of whether it obtains a license. In accordance with Sec. 221, the section requires that the licensure of health professionals employed at Indian entities not be taken into account when determining if a facility meets licensure standards if the health professional is licensed in another state. The section also prohibits IHS, IT, TOs and providers at these facilities from receiving payment or reimbursement from a federal health care program if the facility or provider has been excluded for participation in a federal health program or if the facility or provider's state license has been suspended or revoked. The section defines the term "Federal health care program" and cross-references SSA Sec. 1139 relating to nondiscrimination against providers operated by IHS, an IT, TO, or UIO.

Sec. 157. Access to Federal Insurance

This section adds a new IHCIA Sec. 409 *Access to Federal Insurance* [25 U.S.C. §1647b], which specifies that, notwithstanding 525 U.S.C., an executive order, or an administrative regulation, an IT or TO carrying out programs under ISDEAA or a UIO carrying out programs under IHCIA Title V is entitled to purchase coverage, rights, and benefits for their employees under the Federal Employees Health Benefits Program[29] or the Federal Employees Group Life Insurance program.[30] The section also states that any necessary employee deductions and agency contributions are to be currently deposited in the Employee's Fund applicable to each program.

Sec. 158. Exception for Excepted Benefits

This section adds a new IHCIA Sec. 410 *General Exceptions* [25 U.S.C. §1647c], which directs that the requirements of the previous provisions of IHCIA Title IV of this Act may not apply to certain excepted benefits (involving coverage solely for accidents or disability insurance and certain coverage offered as non-coordinated benefits) defined in Sec. 2791(c) of the PHSA.

Sec. 159. Navajo Nation Medicaid Agency Feasibility Study

This section adds a new IHCIA Sec. 411 *Navajo Nation Medicaid Agency Feasibility Study* [25 U.S.C. §1647d], which requires the Secretary to conduct a study to determine the feasibility of treating the Navajo Nation[31] as a state for Medicaid purposes, for Indians living within the Navajo Nation's boundaries. The provision requires the Secretary to consider the feasibility of certain options and to report the results of the study to specified committees of Congress not later than three years after enactment.

Subtitle E — Health Services for Urban Indians

Subtitle E amends IHCIA Title V, which includes sections related to UIOs and services for urban Indians. Although IHS provides services primarily to American Indians and Alaska Natives living on or near reservations, more than half of this population reside in urban areas.[32] Programs funded under IHCIA Title V seek to make IHS more accessible and available to urban Indians.

There are 34 Urban Indian Health Programs (UIHPs). UIHPs may serve a wider range of eligible persons than the general IHS health care programs, such as members of terminated or state- recognized tribes and their children and grandchildren. These 34 UIHPs operate at 41 locations, with different programs offering different services, such as ambulatory health care, health promotion and education, immunizations, case management, child abuse prevention and treatment, and behavioral health services.[33] In addition to IHS grants and contracts, UIHPs receive funding from state and private sources, patient fees,[34] Medicaid, Medicare, and other non-IHS federal programs.[35]

PPACA maintains and amends existing IHCIA Title V sections and includes new sections that, for example, create new requirements for the Secretary to confer with UIOs, authorize the use of Community Health Representatives program (see IHCIA Title I, Section 109), and expand access to health information technology (HIT).

Sec. 161. Facilities Renovation

This section amends IHCIA Sec. 509 [25 U.S.C. §1659] to permit funds authorized under this section to be used by UIOs for the construction and expansion of facilities. Previously, funds authorized under this section could only be used to make minor renovations to facilities to meet or maintain the standards of the Joint Commission for Accreditation of Health Care Organizations (JCAHO).[36]

Sec. 162. Treatment of Certain Demonstration Projects

This section amends IHCIA Sec. 513 [25 U.S.C. §1660c] to require that the Oklahoma City and Tulsa demonstration projects in Oklahoma (1) be permanent programs within IHS's direct care program; (2) continue to be treated as IHS service units and operating units in the allocation of resources and coordination of care; (3) continue to meet the requirements and definitions of UIOs under this Act; and (4) not be subject to ISDEAA.

Sec. 163. Requirements to Confer with Urban Indian Organizations

This section adds a new IHCIA Sec. 514 *Conferring with Urban Indian Organizations* [25 U.S.C. §1660d], which requires the Secretary to ensure that IHS confers or conferences with UIOs to the greatest extent practicable. It defines "confer" and "conference."

This section also amends IHCIA Sec. 502 [25 U.S.C. §1652] to require the Secretary, under authority of the Snyder Act, to enter into contracts with or make grants to UIOs to establish in urban centers programs that meet the requirements of IHCIA Title V. In addition, the section requires the Secretary, acting through IHS and subject to IHCIA Section 506, to include within grants and contracts any conditions necessary to effect the purpose of IHCIA Title V.

Sec. 164. Expanded Program Authority for Urban Indian Organizations

This section adds a new IHCIA Sec. 515 *Expanded Program Authority for Urban Indian Organizations* [25 U.S.C. §1660e] to authorize the Secretary, acting through IHS, to establish programs, including grants, for UIOs that are identical to programs established pursuant to IHCIA Sec. 218 (prevention of communicable diseases), Sec. 702 (behavioral health prevention and treatment services), and Sec. 708(g) (youth multidrug abuse program).

Sec. 165. Community Health Representatives

This section adds a new IHCIA Sec. 516 *Community Health Representatives* [25 U.S.C. §1660f], which authorizes the Secretary to contract with or make grants to UIOs for the employment of Indians trained as health service providers through the Community Health Representatives Program under IHCIA Section 109.

Sec. 166. Use of Federal Government Facilities and Sources of Supply; HIT

This section adds a new IHCIA Sec. 517 *Use of Federal Government Facilities and Sources of Supply* [25 U.S.C. §1660g], which authorizes the Secretary to (1) permit UIOs carrying out contracts or grants under this title to use existing HHS facilities and equipment; (2) donate excess IHS or General Services Administration real or personal property to such organizations; and (3) acquire excess or surplus federal government real or personal property for donation to such organizations (subject to a priority for tribes and tribal organizations). The section permits UIOs carrying out contracts or grants under this title to be deemed to be federal executive agencies under Section 201 of the Federal Property and Administrative Services Act of 1949, with access to federal prime vendors, when the organizations are carrying out IHCIA Title V contracts or grants.

This section also adds a new IHCIA Sec. 518 *Health Information Technology* [25 U.S.C. §1660h], which authorizes the Secretary to make grants to UIOs under this title for the development, adoption, and implementation of HIT (as defined in PHSA Section 3000, telemedicine services development, and related infrastructure).

Subtitle F — Organizational Improvements

Subtitle F amends IHCIA Title VI. The title established IHS 's organizational position as part of the PHS within HHS. PPACA reaffirms IHS's position in the PHS and establishes that the Director of IHS reports directly to the Secretary. PPACA also establishes an Office of Direct Service Tribes within IHS to address the needs of tribes that receive services administered by IHS as opposed to services administered by an IT or a TO under contract or compact (these are called direct service tribes). In addition, PPACA requires a plan for a new area office for tribes located in Nevada. Under the current IHS organization, tribes in Nevada receive services through the Phoenix Area Office.

Sec. 171. Establishment of the IHS as an Agency of the Public Health Service

This section amends IHCIA Sec. 601 [25 U.S.C. §1661]. It maintains IHS's position within the PHS, and maintains language establishing the IHS Director as an official appointed by the President with the advice and consent of the Senate for a four-year term. This section also amends IHCIA Sec. 601 to state that the IHS Director reports to the Secretary and the incumbent at enactment will remain as Director. The section specifies that the position of the Director reports directly to the Secretary on all policy and budget matters related to Indian health, interacts with assistant secretaries and agency heads on Indian health, and coordinates department activities on Indian health. The section maintains Indian preference for IHS employment.

Sec. 172. Office of Direct Service Tribes

This section adds a new IHCIA Sec. 603 *Office of Direct Service Tribes* [25 U.S.C. §1663], which establishes an Office of Direct Service Tribes within the office of the IHS Director. The section also specifies the responsibilities of the new office, including providing leadership, guidance and support within IHS for direct service tribes, specified consultation responsibilities, and others.

Sec. 173. Nevada Area Office

This section adds a new IHCIA Sec. 604 *Nevada Area Office* [25 U.S.C. §1663a], which requires the Secretary, in a manner consistent with IHS consultation policy, to submit to Congress, within one year of enactment, a plan to create a new Nevada Area Office distinct from the current Phoenix Area Office. If the Secretary fails to submit a plan, then the Secretary is required to withhold operation funds (as defined) from the IHS Office of the Director provided that such withholding does not adversely impact IHS health services. Withheld funds could be restored at the discretion of the Secretary when the plan is submitted.

Subtitle G—Behavioral Health Programs

Subtitle G amends IHCIA Title VII "Behavioral Health Programs," which includes sections that authorize behavioral health care programs. PPACA replaced the existing Title VII with new language that authorizes programs to create a "comprehensive behavioral health prevention and treatment program" providing a "continuum of behavioral health care" (see IHCIA Sections 701 and 703 of Sec. 181 below). PPACA also creates a new subsection of Title VII that authorizes new programs focused on preventing youth suicide.

Sec. 181. Behavioral Health Programs

This section replaces IHCIA Title VII with the following new programs:

Subtitle A—General Programs

Sec. 701. Definitions

This section adds a new Sec. 701 *Definitions* [25 U.S.C. §1665], which defines a number of terms used in the title, including "Alcohol-related neurodevelopmental disorders," "dual diagnosis," "FAS or fetal alcohol syndrome," "rehabilitation," and "substance abuse."

Sec. 702. Behavioral Health Prevention and Treatment Services

This section adds a new Sec. 702 *Behavioral Health Prevention and Treatment Service*[25 U.S.C. §1665 a]. The section includes the purpose of the title, which includes directing the Secretary, acting through IHS, to develop a comprehensive behavioral health care program that emphasizes collaboration among alcohol and substance abuse, social services, and mental health programs. The section also requires the Secretary to encourage ITs, TOs, and UIOs to develop tribal, local, and area-wide plans for Indian behavioral health services that include assessments of specified behavioral problems, the number of Indians affected, the financial and human costs, the existing and necessary resources to prevent and treat such problems, and an estimate of necessary funding. The section requires the Secretary to coordinate with existing national clearinghouses to include such plans and any reports on their outcomes; ensure access to the plans and outcomes by IHS, ITs, TOs, and UIOs; and provide technical assistance in the development of these plans and related standards of care. The section also requires the Secretary to provide, through IHS, and to the extent feasible and funded, a comprehensive continuum of behavioral health care, as well as specified services for Indian children, adults, families, and elders. The section authorizes ITs, TOs, and UIOs to establish community behavioral health plans, requires IHS and BIA cooperation and assistance in developing and implementing such plans, and authorizes grants to ITs and TOs for technical assistance and administrative support for such plans. The section requires the Secretary, through IHS, ITs, TOs, and UIOs, to coordinate behavioral health planning with other federal and state agencies. The section also requires the Secretary, within one year of enactment, to assess the need, availability, and cost for inpatient mental health care and facilities for Indians, including possible conversion of existing, underused IHS hospital beds into psychiatric units.

Sec. 703. Memoranda of Agreement with the Department of Interior

This section adds a new IHCIA Sec. 703 *Memoranda of Agreement with the Department of Interior* [25 U.S.C. §1665b], which requires the Secretary and the Secretary of the Interior, not later than 12 months after enactment, to develop and enter into memoranda of agreement, or update the memoranda of agreement required by Sec. 4205 of the Indian Alcohol and Substance Abuse Prevention and Treatment Act.[37] The section specifies that the memoranda of agreement must address eight specified activities, including a comprehensive assessment and coordination of mental health care needs and services available or unavailable to Indians, and the ensuring and protection of Indians' right of access to general mental health services. The section further requires that the memoranda include provisions assigning to IHS responsibility for determining the scope of alcohol and substance abuse problems among Indians, assessing existing and needed resources, and estimating necessary funding. The section also requires that each memorandum, renewal, or modification be published in the *Federal Register*, with copies to ITs, TOs, and UIOs.

Sec. 704. Behavioral Health Prevention and Treatment Program

This section adds a new Sec. 704 *Comprehensive Behavioral Health Prevention and Treatment Program* [25 U.S.C. §1665c], which requires the Secretary to provide, through IHS, a program of comprehensive behavioral health, prevention, treatment, and aftercare, for Indian tribal members that includes education, specified treatments, rehabilitation, training, and diagnostic services. The section authorizes the Secretary, through IHS, to provide the services through contracts with public and private behavioral health providers, and requires the Secretary to assist ITs and TOs with developing criteria for certification of providers and accreditation of facilities.

Sec. 705. Mental Health Technician Program

This section adds a new Sec. 705 *Mental Health Technician Program* [25 U.S.C. §1665d], which requires the Secretary, under the Snyder Act, to establish within IHS a mental health technician training and employment program for Indians. The section also requires the Secretary, through IHS, to provide high-standard paraprofessional training in mental health care, to supervise and evaluate these technicians, and to ensure that the program includes using and promoting traditional Indian health care practices of the tribes served.

Sec. 706. Licensing Requirement for Mental Health Care Workers

This section adds a new Sec. 706 *Licensing Requirement for Mental Health Care Workers* [25 U.S.C. §1665e], which, subject to IHCIA Sec. 221 (regarding licensing), requires that any person employed as a psychologist, social worker, or marriage and family therapist to provide mental health care services to Indians in a clinic be licensed to provide the specified service. The section also provides that a trainee in psychology, social work, or marriage and family therapy may provide mental health care services if the trainee is directly supervised by someone licensed in the specified service, is enrolled in or has completed at least two years of course work in an accredited post-secondary education program for the specified service, and meets other requirements that the Secretary may establish.

Sec. 707. Indian Women Treatment Programs

This section adds a new Sec. 707 *Indian Women Treatment Programs* [25 U.S.C. §1665f], which authorizes the Secretary, consistent with IHCIA Sec. 701, to make grants to ITs, TOs, and UIOs to develop and implement a comprehensive behavioral health program for prevention, intervention, treatment, and relapse prevention that specifically addresses the cultural, historical, social, and childcare needs of Indian women. The section specifies uses of the grants, including community training and education, counseling, support, and development of prevention and intervention models. The section also requires the Secretary, in consultation with ITs and TOs, to establish grant approval criteria, and to allocate 20% of the program's funds for grants to UIOs.

Sec. 708. Indian Youth Program

This section adds a new Sec. 708 *Indian Youth Program* [25 U.S.C. §1665g], which establishes a number of Indian youth behavioral health programs. The section requires the Secretary, consistent with IHCIA Sec. 701, to develop and implement a program for acute detoxification and treatment for Indian youth, including behavioral health services, regional treatment centers with detoxification and rehabilitation services, and local programs developed by ITs or TOs under ISDEAA. The section requires the Secretary, through IHS, to construct, renovate, or purchase, and staff and operate (under the Snyder Act) at least one youth regional treatment center or treatment network in each IHS area (treating the California Area as two areas), in a location agreed upon by a majority of the area's tribes; the section also authorizes funding to two specified Alaska Native entities for youth treatment facilities in Alaska.[38] The section authorizes the Secretary to provide intermediate behavioral health services for Indian children and adolescents, and specifies that such services include pretreatment assistance; inpatient, outpatient, and aftercare services; emergency care; suicide prevention; and prevention and treatment of mental illness and dysfunctional and self-destructive behavior, including child abuse and family violence. The section sets the allowable uses of funds for intermediate behavioral health services, and requires the Secretary, in consultation with ITs and TOs, to develop grant approval criteria.

The section also requires the Secretary, in consultation with ITs and TOs, to identify and use suitable federally owned structures for local residential or regional behavioral health treatment for Indian youths, and establish suitability guidelines. The section allows the use of any such federally owned structure under terms agreed upon by the Secretary, the responsible federal agency, and the IT or TO operating the program. The section also requires the Secretary, ITs, and TOs, in cooperation with the Secretary of Interior, to develop local community-based rehabilitation and aftercare services provided by trained staff in each IHS service unit for Indian youths with significant behavioral health problems, including long-term treatment, community reintegration, and monitoring. The section requires the Secretary, in providing services under this section, to provide for inclusion of family in such services, and specifies that not less than 10% of funds for the local rehabilitation and aftercare services program may be used for outpatient care of adult family members of an Indian youth in the program. The section also requires the Secretary, through IHS, to provide programs and services to prevent and treat multi-drug abuse among Indian youths in Indian communities, on or near reservations, and in urban areas, and provide appropriate mental health services. The section requires the Secretary to collect data on specified aspects of Indian youth mental health for the report under IHCIA Sec. 801.

Sec. 709. Mental Health Facilities Design, Construction, and Staffing

This section adds a new Sec. 709 *Inpatient and Community-Based Mental Health Facilities Design, Construction, and Staffing* [25 U.S.C. §1665h], which authorizes the Secretary, through IHS, to provide in each IHS area, not later than one year after enactment, at least one inpatient mental health facility for Indians with behavioral health problems. The section requires that California be considered two areas and requires the Secretary to consider the conversion of existing underused IHS hospital beds into psychiatric units to meet the need for such facilities.

Sec. 710. Training and Community Education

This section adds a new Sec. 710 *Training and Community Education* [25 U.S.C. §1665i], which requires the Secretary, in cooperation with the Secretary of the Interior, to develop and implement in each IHS service unit or tribal program a program of community education and involvement for specified tribal community leaders in behavioral health issues, possibly including community-based training, or to assist tribes and tribal organizations in doing so. The section requires the Secretary to provide specified instruction in behavioral health issues to appropriate IHS and BIA employees and personnel in contracted IHS and BIA programs and schools.[39] In addition, this section requires the Secretary, as part of the community education and employee instruction programs, to develop and provide community-based training models addressing specified aspects of behavioral health problems, in consultation with ITs, TOs, and Indian alcohol and substance abuse prevention experts.

Sec. 711. Behavioral Health Program

This section adds a new Sec. 711 *Behavioral Health Program* [25 U.S.C. §1665j], which authorizes the Secretary, through IHS, to develop and implement programs to deliver innovative community-based behavioral health services to Indians, and authorize grants to ITs and TOs for such programs. The section specifies criteria for awarding such grants, and requires the Secretary to use the same criteria in evaluating all project applications.

Sec. 712. Fetal Alcohol Spectrum Disorder Programs

This section adds a new Sec. 712 *Fetal Alcohol Spectrum Disorders Programs* [25 U.S.C. §1665k], which authorizes the Secretary, through IHS, to develop and implement fetal alcohol disorder (FAD) programs (as defined in IHCIA Sec. 4), consistent with IHCIA Sec. 701, and to establish criteria for approval of funding applications. The section specifies grant uses, including developing and providing services for the prevention, intervention, treatment, and aftercare for those affected by FAD; early childhood intervention projects; supportive services; and housing. The section requires the Secretary, through IHS, to provide FAD prevention, treatment, and aftercare services as well as specified support services.

The section also requires the Secretary to make grants through the Substance Abuse and Mental Health Services Administration (SAMHSA) in HHS to ITs, TOs, and UIOs for applied research projects to elevate the understanding of methods to prevent, intervene, treat, or provide rehabilitation and aftercare for Indians affected by fetal alcohol spectrum disorders. The section requires that 10% of appropriations under this section be used for grants to UIOs funded under IHCIA Title V.

Sec. 713. Child Sexual Abuse Prevention and Treatment Programs

This section adds a new Sec. 713 *Child Sexual Abuse Prevention and Treatment Programs* [25 U.S.C. §1665l], which requires the Secretary, through IHS, and consistent with IHCIA Sec. 701, to establish in every IHS Area treatment programs for child victims of sexual abuse who are Indians or members of Indian households. The section requires four uses of funding, including developing community education, identifying and providing treatment to victims, and developing culturally sensitive prevention models and diagnostic tools. The section requires that the programs be carried out in coordination with programs and services authorized under the Indian Child Protection and Family Violence Prevention Act.[40]

Sec. 714. Domestic and Sexual Violence Prevention and Treatment

This section adds a new Sec. 714 *Domestic and Sexual Violence Prevention and Treatment* [25 U.S.C. §1665m], which authorizes the Secretary to establish programs in each IHS Area to prevent and treat Indian victims of domestic violence or sexual violence. The section requires that program funds be used for prevention and community education programs, behavioral health services and medical treatment for victims (including examinations by sexual assault nurse examiners), rape kits, and development of prevention and intervention models (including traditional health care). The section requires the Secretary to establish protocols, policies, procedures, standards, training curricula, and training and certification requirements for victim services within one year of enactment, and requires a report on these activities to specified committees of Congress within 18 months of enactment. The section also requires the Secretary, in coordination with the Attorney General (AG), federal and tribal law enforcement agencies, IHPs, and victim organizations, to develop victim services and victim advocate training programs, for specified purposes, and it requires the Secretary, within two years of enactment, to report to specified committees of Congress on such services and programs, including improvements, obstacles, costs needed to address the obstacles, and any recommendations.

Sec. 715. Behavioral Health Research

This section adds a new Sec. 715 *Behavioral Health Research* [25 U.S.C. §1665n], which requires the Secretary, in consultation with appropriate federal agencies, to make contracts with or grants to ITs, TOs, and UIOs, and appropriate institutions for research on the incidence and prevalence of behavioral health problems among Indians served by IHS, ITs, or TOs and in urban areas. The section directs that research priorities include the multifactorial causes of Indian youth suicide; the interrelationship of behavioral health problems with alcoholism, suicide, homicide, and family violence, especially on children; and the development of models of prevention techniques, especially in regard to children.

Subtitle B—Indian Youth Suicide Services

Sec. 721. Findings and Purpose

This section adds a new Sec. 721 *Findings and Purpose* [25 U.S.C. §1667], which includes the findings and the stated purposes of this section, which are (1) to authorize the Secretary to carry out a demonstration project to test the use of telemental health services in suicide prevention, intervention, and treatment of Indian youth (through specified means); (2) to encourage ITs, TOs, and other mental health care providers serving residents of Indian country to obtain the services of predoctoral psychology and psychiatry interns; and (3) to enhance the provision of mental health care services to Indian youth through existing SAMHSA grants.

Sec. 722. Definitions

This section adds a new Sec. 722 *Definitions* [25 U.S.C. §1667a], which defines the following terms: "Administration," "demonstration project," and "telemental health."

Sec. 723. Indian Youth Telemental Health Demonstration Project

This section adds a new Sec. 723 *Indian Youth Telemental Health Demonstration Project* [25 U.S.C. §1667b], which authorizes the Secretary to carry out a demonstration project by making four-year grants to not more than five ITs and TOs with telehealth capabilities to use for telemental health services in youth suicide prevention and treatment. The section defines terms and directs the Secretary to give priority to ITs and TOs that serve tribal communities that have a demonstrated need or are isolated and have limited access to mental health services, that enter into collaborative partnerships to provide the services, or that operate a detention facility where youth are detained. The section describes the uses of the grants, including the use of telemedicine for psychotherapy, psychiatric assessments, and diagnostic interviews of Indian youth; the provision of clinical expertise and other medical advice to frontline health care providers working with Indian youth; training and related support for community leaders, family members, and health and education workers who work with Indian youth; the development of culturally relevant educational materials on suicide prevention and intervention; data collection and reporting; and the use of the tribe's traditional health care practices. The section includes requirements for grant applications, encourages collaboration among grantees and grantee reports to the national clearinghouse under IHCIA Sec. 701, and requires grantees to submit annual reports to the Secretary. In addition, the section requires the Secretary to submit a report to specified committees of Congress no later than 270 days after termination of the demonstration project. The report must include evaluations of whether the project should be made permanent or expanded to more than five grants and to UIOs. The section authorizes appropriations of such sums as may be necessary to carry out this section.

Sec. 724. SAMHSA Grants

This section adds a new Sec. 724 *Substance Abuse and Mental Health Services Administration Grants* [25 U.S.C. §1667c], which requires the Secretary to streamline the process by which ITs and TOs could apply for SAMHSA grants, including providing non-electronic methods. For SAMHSA grants for activities relating to mental health, suicide prevention, or suicide-related risk factors, and for which an IT or TO is eligible, in order to fulfill the trust responsibility of the United States to ITs, the Secretary is required to consider the needs of ITs or TOs that serve populations with documented high suicide rates, regardless of whether those ITs or TOs possess adequate personnel or infrastructure to fulfill all applicable grant requirements. Notwithstanding any other provision of law, no IT or TO is required to apply for SAMHSA grants through a state or state agency. Any state applying for a SAMHSA grant based on statewide data is required to consider the Indian population within the state and make reasonable efforts to collaborate with ITs within the state in implementing SAMHSA grant programs. ITs and TOs are not required to provide non-federal contributions for any SAMHSA grant. The

Secretary is also required to conduct outreach to rural and isolated tribes to promote the purposes of this subtitle. The Secretary is required to take other measures to assure access to mental health and suicide prevention services by ITs at high risk, as defined by suicide rates, socioeconomic status, and other factors. The section also authorizes to be appropriated such sums as may be necessary to carry out this section. Finally, the Secretary is required to ensure that any recipient of a grant under PHSA Sec. 520E (grants for youth suicide prevention and early intervention strategies that are not exclusive to tribal awardees) provides training to those serving Indian youth under the grant program in the recognition of suicide risk among Indian youth.

Sec. 725 Use of Predoctoral Psychology and Psychiatry Interns

This section adds a new Sec. 725 *Use of Predoctoral Psychology and Psychiatry Interns* [25 U.S.C. §1667d], which requires the Secretary to carry out activities to encourage ITs, TOs, and other mental health care providers to obtain the services of predoctoral psychology and psychiatry interns in order to increase the quantity of patients served by those providers, and for purposes of recruitment and retention.

Sec. 726. Indian Youth Life Skills Demonstration Program

This section adds a new Sec. 726 *Indian Youth Life Skills Development Demonstration Program* [25 U.S.C. §1667e], which authorizes the Secretary, through SAMHSA, to carry out a demonstration program to test the effectiveness of a culturally compatible, school-based, life skills curriculum for the prevention of American Indian and Alaska Native adolescent suicide. The program may use tribal partnerships, assistance from SAMHSA, training, advisory councils, and other approaches. The section also authorizes the Secretary to award demonstration grants to ITs, TOs, or other authorized entities or partnerships who meet specified application requirements, to implement the life skills curriculum. Not more than five grants may be awarded for terms of not less than four years, and at least one grant must be awarded to each of (1) a school operated by the Bureau of Indian Education (BIE); (2) a Tribal school; and (3) a school receiving payments under Sec. 8002 or 8003 of the Elementary and Secondary Education Act of 1965. Grant funds may be used for a number of specific activities. The Secretary is also required to conduct annual program evaluations, and to report to Congress regarding the program within 180 days of its termination, following a public comment period. The section authorizes an appropriation of $1 million for each of FY2010 through FY2014.

Subtitle H — Miscellaneous

Subtitle H amends IHCIA Title VIII, which includes a number of miscellaneous provisions, including those that require annual reports about activities authorized in IHCIA, and those related to a number of demonstration programs in specified topics and areas. PPACA amends existing sections about certain persons' eligibility for IHS services; adds new sections about medical records; the designation of CHSDAs; IHS budget submissions; monitoring of prescription drugs; required reports; and a variety of other topics.

Sec. 191. Medical Quality Assurance Records Confidentiality

This section adds a new IHCIA Sec. 805 [25 U.S.C. §1675], which makes medical quality assurance records created by an IHP or a UIHP confidential and privileged, and prohibits their disclosure except to specified entities for specified purposes. The section exempts such records from the Freedom of Information Act,[41] requires the Secretary to promulgate regulations, and defines terms.

Sec. 192. Arizona, North Dakota, and South Dakota as CHSDAs

This section amends IHCIA Sec. 808 [25 U.S.C. §1678] with a new section *Arizona as a Contract Health Service Delivery Area* that designates the State of Arizona as an IHS CHSDA for the members of ITs in Arizona. The section also prohibits IHS from curtailing any services as a result of this section.

This section also adds a new IHCIA Sec. 808A *North Dakota and South Dakota as CHSDAs* [25 U.S.C. § 1 678a], which designates North Dakota and South Dakota as one CHSDA for the purpose of providing CHS to members of ITs in these states. This section also prohibits IHS from curtailing any services as a result of this provision.

This section also amends IHCIA Sec. 809 [25 U.S.C. §1679] with a new section *Eligibility of California Indians* that designates specified California Indians as eligible for IHS health services, including members of federally-recognized tribes, descendants of Indians residing in California as of June 1, 1852 (if living in California and meeting other criteria), Indians holding trust interests in certain types of land, and Indians (and their descendants) listed on the plans for asset distribution in California under the Act of August 18, 1958 (terminating recognition of certain California tribes). The section prohibits construing anything in the section as expanding California Indians' eligibility for IHS health services beyond their eligibility as of May 1,1986.

Sec. 193. Methods to Increase Access to Health Professionals

This section adds a new IHCIA Sec. 812 *National Health Service Corps* [25 U.S.C. §1680b], which prohibits the Secretary from removing a member of the National Health Service Corps (NHSC)[42] from an IHP or UIO, or withdrawing funding to support such member, unless the Secretary, acting through the IHS, ensures that Indians will experience no reduction in services. The section also authorizes that, at the IHP 's request, the services of NHSC personnel assigned to an IHP may be limited to the persons eligible for services from such program.

Sec. 194. Health Services for Ineligible Persons

This section amends IHCIA Sec. 813 [25 U.S.C. §1680c] with new language that authorizes IHS health services for certain otherwise ineligible persons, including spouses or children of eligible Indians, non-Indian women carrying Indian babies, or persons in need of emergency stabilization, or for prevention of communicable diseases. The section authorizes the governing body of Indian tribes operating health facilities under ISDEAA contracts to determine whether to provide services to ineligible persons. The section also sets criteria for providing services, such as requiring reimbursement and tribal approval, and directs that reimbursements, including under Medicare or Medicaid, be credited to the facility providing the service and be available for expenditure by the facility. The section permits the Secretary to provide services to indigent individuals who are not otherwise eligible for IHS services provided that the state or local government agrees to reimburse IHS for providing this service. The section also permits extending hospital privileges to non-IHS health care practitioners who provide service to certain ineligible persons.

Sec. 195. Annual Budget Submission

This section adds a new IHCIA Sec. 826 *Annual Budget Submission* [25 U.S.C. §1680p], which requires the President, effective with the submission of the FY20 11 budget, to request amounts that reflect changes in the cost of health care services as adjusted by the consumer price index for inflation, and amounts that reflect changes in the size of the population served by IHS.

Sec. 196. Prescription Drug Monitoring

This sections adds a new IHCIA Sec. 827 *Prescription Drug Monitoring* [25 U.S.C. §1680q], which requires the Secretary, in coordination with the Secretary of the Interior and AG to establish a prescription drug monitoring program, to be carried out at facilities operated by IHS, ITs, TOs, and UIOs. The section also requires the Secretary to submit a report within 18 months of enactment to specified congressional committees describing (1) the prescription drug monitoring program needs of facilities operated by IHS, ITs, TOs, and UIOs; (2) the planned development and the means to carry out a prescription drug monitoring program, including relevant statutory or administrative limitations; and (3) the need for coordination with any state prescription drug monitoring program. The section requires the AG, in conjunction with the Secretary and the Secretary of the Interior, to conduct (1) an assessment of the capacity of, and support required by, relevant federal and tribal agencies to collect and analyze data and exchange information regarding incidents of prescription drug abuse in Indian communities and exchange information regarding prescription drug abuse in Indian communities; and (2) training for Indian health care providers, tribal leaders, law enforcement, and school officials regarding awareness and prevention of prescription drug abuse and strategies to improve and address prescription drug abuse in Indian communities. The section also requires the AG, within 18 months of enactment, to submit a report to specified congressional committees that describes certain factors regarding the AG's responsibilities related to prescription drug abuse in Indian communities.

Sec. 197. Tribal Health Program Option for Cost Sharing

This section adds a new IHCIA Sec. 828 *Tribal Health Program Option for Cost Sharing* [25 U.S.C. §1680r], which states that nothing in IHCIA limits the ability of a THP operating any health program, service, function, activity, or facility funded in whole or in part by IHS through a compact with IHS under Title V of the ISDEAA, to charge an Indian for services provided by the THP. The section also states that nothing in IHCIA authorizes IHS to charge an Indian for services or to require a THP to charge an Indian for services.

Sec. 198. Disease and Injury Prevention Reports

This section adds a new IHCIA Sec. 829 *Disease and Injury Prevention* [25 U.S.C. §1680s], which requires the Secretary to submit, within 18 months of enactment, a report to specified congressional committees describing all disease and injury prevention activities conducted by IHS either independently or in conjunction with federal departments, agencies, and ITs, and the effectiveness of such activities.

Sec. 199. Other GAO Reports

This section adds new IHCIA Sec. 830 *Other GAO Reports* [25 U.S.C. §1680t], which requires two specified GAO reports to be submitted to Congress within 18 months of enactment. GAO must conduct studies on (1) the effectiveness of the coordination of health care services provided to Indians: (a) through Medicare, Medicaid, or CHIP; (b) by IHS; or (c) by using funds provided by state or local governments or ITs; and (2) the use of CHS including analyses of amounts reimbursed to providers, suppliers, and entities under CHS, compared to reimbursements through other public and private programs; barriers to access to health care under CHS; adequacy of federal funding of CHS; and other matters GAO determines appropriate. This study must be conducted in consultation with IHS, ITs, and TOs, and must include recommendations on appropriate federal funding for CHS and ways to use such funding efficiently.

Sec. 200. Traditional Health Care Practices

This section adds a new IHCIA Sec. 831 *Traditional Health Care Practices* [25 U.S.C. §1680u], which states that the United States is not liable for damage, injuries, or death that may result from traditional health care practices, consistent with IHS standards for the provision of health care, health promotion, and disease prevention provided pursuant to IHCIA (although the Secretary may promote traditional health care practices). The section further specifies that nothing in the section may be construed to alter any liability of other obligation that the United States has under ISDEAA.

Sec. 201. Director of HIV/AIDS Prevention and Treatment

This section adds a new IHCIA Sec. 832 *Director of HIV/AIDS Prevention and Treatment* [25 U.S.C. §1680v], which requires the Secretary, acting through IHS, to establish within IHS a Director of HIV/AIDS Prevention and Treatment. The Director is required to (1) coordinate and promote HIV/AIDS prevention and treatment activities for Indians; (2) provide technical assistance to ITs, TOs, and UIOs regarding existing HIV/AIDS prevention and treatment programs; and (3) ensure interagency coordination to facilitate the inclusion of Indians in federal HIV/AIDS research and grant opportunities with an emphasis on programs operated under the Ryan White Comprehensive AIDS Resource Emergency Act of 1990 and its amendments. The section also requires that, not later than two years after enactment and every two years thereafter, the Director submit to Congress a report describing the activities carried out under this section and the Director's findings related to HIV/AIDS prevention and treatment activities specific to Indians.

Sec. 10221(b)(3) Abortion Funding Restrictions

This section amends IHCIA Sec. 806 [25 U.S.C. § 1676] to state that any funds appropriated to HHS may not be used for the performance or coverage of abortion. In addition, the section states that any limitation included in another federal law with respect to the performance or coverage of abortion also applies to funds appropriated to IHS.

TITLE II—AMENDMENTS TO OTHER ACTS[43]

Title II of the Indian Health Care Improvement Reauthorization and Extension Act, as enacted, contains one provision that amends and reauthorizes the Native Hawaiian Health Care Act of 1988 (NHHCA, P.L. 100-579, as amended; 42 25 U.S.C. §11701-11714),which authorizes health education, health promotion, disease prevention services, and health professions scholarship programs for Native Hawaiians.[44]

Sec. 202. Reauthorization of Native Hawaiian Health Care Programs

This section reauthorizes expired appropriations authorities in the NHHCA [42 U.S.C. § 11701- 117 14] through FY2019. This section also amends the NHHCA [42 U.S.C. § 11705], effective on December 5, 2006, to permit a specified private educational organization (Kamehameha Schools Bishop Estate) identified in Sec. 7202(16) of the Elementary and Secondary Education Act of 1965 [20 U.S.C.75 12(16)] to continue to offer educational programs and services to Native Hawaiians (as defined in that Act) first, and to other groups only after the needs of Native Hawaiians have been met. This section also amends the definition of "health promotion" in NHHCA Sec. 12(2).

APPENDIX A. TIMELINE OF IHCIA PROVISIONS IN PPACA

In some instances, PPACA, specifies dates for key administrative or programmatic activities or requirements. The following timeline (see **Table A-1**) lists the provisions summarized in this report that include dates, such as those that include dates for reports.

Other activities or requirements that have no date specified in PPACA and are implicitly effective upon enactment (March 23, 2010) are not included in this timeline. All activities authorized in the IHCIA are discretionary and subject to appropriations by Congress. Given this, all deadlines below may not be considered binding since they are subject to appropriated funds.

Table A-1 lists the PPACA dates, which are grouped by subtitle in the IHCIA Reauthorization and Extension Act of 2009. Not all subtitles are included, as some subtitles do not include provisions with specified deadlines. Within each subtitle, table entries are organized with key dates in chronological order. Effective dates stated in terms of days, months, or years after enactment have been converted to calendar dates (e.g., 180 days is 9/19/2010; six months is 9/23/2010, etc.). Table entries for specific implementation requirements or deadlines that are not tied to a specific calendar date are presented at the end of each title. Each table entry includes the IHCIA Reauthorization and Extension Act section number as enacted by Section 10221 of PPACA; a descriptive title for each activity or requirement; a brief description of the activity or requirement; and the associated start date, or effective date. Where applicable, frequency or duration associated with specific activities or requirements is noted. All of IHCIA Title VII is amended by Section 181 of the IHCIA Reauthorization and Extension Act; therefore, for requirements contained in Section 181 the subsection of IHCIA Title VII it amends is noted in parentheses.

For additional information on provisions that appear in the timeline, refer to the more detailed section summaries in the report. For definitions of acronyms used in the timeline, refer to Appendix B. Unless otherwise stated, references in the table to "the Secretary" refer to the Secretary of Health and Human Services (HHS).

Table A-1. Timeline of IHCIA Provisions in PPACA

Section of the IHCIA Reauthorization and Extension Act of 2009 as enacted by PPACA Sec. 10221	Title	Description	Start or Effective Date or Deadline
Subtitle B–Health Services			
Sec. 127	Behavioral Training and Community Education Programs	Requires the Secretary to develop a plan to increase behavioral health services by creating 500 additional staff positions within 5 years of enactment.	6/21/2010
Sec. 136	Office of Indian Men's Health	Requires the Secretary, through IHS, to submit a report to Congress describing the activities carried out by the Office of Indian Men's Health and findings related to Indian Men's Health.	3/23/2012
Sec. 133	Prevention and Control of Communicable Diseases	Requires the Secretary to submit a biennial report to Congress on the grants awarded for the prevention, control, and elimination of communicable and infectious diseases.	3/23/2012
Sec. 121	Indian Health Care Improvement Fund	Requires the Secretary to submit a report to Congress on the current health status and resource deficiencies of each tribe or service unit.	3/23/2013
Sec. 137	CHS Administration and Disbursement Formula	Requires GAO to submit a report to Congress describing the results of a study about the CHS program including funding levels and administration of the program.	As soon as practicable after enactment

Section of the IHCIA Reauthorization and Extension Act of 2009 as enacted by PPACA Sec. 10221	Title	Description	Start or Effective Date or Deadline
Subtitle C–Health Facilities			
Sec. 141	Health Care Facilities Priority System	Requires the Secretary, in the annual report required in Sec. 801, to submit a report to the President describing the health care facility priority system and the top 10 priorities for various construction projects under this priority system.	February 7, 2011[a]
Sec. 141	Health Care Facilities Priority System	Requires the Secretary to submit an initial report to Congress with a ranked list of all IHS, IT, and TO health care facility needs. Further requires the Secretary to submit an updated version of this report every 5 years beginning in 2011.	3/23/2011
Sec. 141	Health Care Facilities Priority System	Requires GAO to study the methodologies used by IHS to develop its health care priority system.	One year after new priority system is developed
Sec. 147	Mobile Health Station Demonstration Program	Requires the Secretary to submit a report to Congress that describes and evaluates the results of a demonstration project establishing mobile health stations.	One year after the demonstration program is established

Table A-1. (Continued)

Section of the IHCIA Reauthorization and Extension Act of 2009 as enacted by PPACA Sec. 10221	Title	Description	Start or Effective Date or Deadline
Subtitle D–Access to Health Services			
Sec. 159	Navajo Nation Medicaid Agency Feasibility Study	Requires the Secretary to submit a report to Congress considering the feasibility of considering the Navajo Nation a state for Medicaid purposes.	3/23/2013
Subtitle F–Organizational Improvements			
Sec. 173	Nevada Area Office	Requires the Secretary to submit a plan to Congress to create a new Nevada Area Office.	3/23/2011
Subtitle G–Behavioral Health Programs			
Sec. 181 (Sec. 702)	Behavioral Health Prevention and Treatment Services	Requires the Secretary, acting through IHS, to assess the need, availability, and cost of inpatient mental health care for Indians.	3/23/2011
Sec. 181 (Sec. 703)	Memoranda of Agreement with the Department of the Interior	Requires the Secretary, acting through IHS, and the Secretary of the Interior to develop and enter into a memorandum of agreement regarding mental illness and self-destructive behavior among Indians and strategies to address unmet needs.	3/23/2011
Sec. 181 (Sec. 714)	Domestic and Sexual Violence Prevention and Treatment	Requires the Secretary to establish protocols, policies, procedures, and programs for victims of domestic or sexual violence.	3/23/2011

Section of the IHCIA Reauthorization and Extension Act of 2009 as enacted by PPACA Sec. 10221	Title	Description	Start or Effective Date or Deadline
Sec. 181 (Sec. 714)	Domestic and Sexual Violence Prevention and Treatment	Requires the Secretary to submit a report to Congress on protocols, policies, procedures, and other programs for victims of domestic or sexual violence.	9/23/2011
Sec. 181 (Sec. 714)	Domestic and Sexual Violence Prevention and Treatment	Requires the Secretary to submit a report to Congress on domestic and sexual violence prevention and treatment programs, The report should also include improvement needed, obstacles faced, and costs of addressing these obstacles.	3/23/2012
Sec. 181 (Sec. 726)	Indian Youth Life Skills Demonstration Program	Requires the Secretary to report on the results of a program evaluation conducted on a demonstration program to test the effectiveness of programs to prevent American Indian and Alaska Native suicide.	180 days after the termination of the demonstration program and after the public comment period.
Subtitle H–Miscellaneous			
Sec. 195	Annual Budget Submission	Requires the President to include, within the IHS annual budget request and justification, amounts that reflect changes in the cost of health care services adjusted by the consumer price index and amounts adjusted to reflect changes in the IHS service population.	February 1, 2010[b]

Table A-1. (Continued)

Section of the IHCIA Reauthorization and Extension Act of 2009 as enacted by PPACA Sec. 10221	Title	Description	Start or Effective Date or Deadline
Sec. 196	Prescription Drug Monitoring	Requires the Secretary to submit a report describing the specified elements of the prescription drug monitoring program.	9/23/2011
Sec. 196	Prescription Drug Monitoring	Requires the AG to submit a report to Congress describing certain factors regarding the AG's responsibility related to prescription drug abuse in Indian communities.	9/23/2011
Sec. 198	Disease and Injury Prevention Reports	Requires the Secretary to submit a report to Congress describing disease and injury prevention activities by IHS and other federal agencies.	9/23/2011
Sec. 199	Other GAO Reports	Requires GAO to submit a report to Congress containing the results and recommendations resulting from a study evaluating the effectiveness of the coor-dination of health care services provided to Indians either through Medicare, Medicaid, or CHIP, with those provided by IHS, with funding from state or local governments or ITs.	9/23/2011

Section of the IHCIA Reauthorization and Extension Act of 2009 as enacted by PPACA Sec. 10221	Title	Description	Start or Effective Date or Deadline
Sec. 199	Other GAO Reports	Requires the Comptroller General to study (in consultation with IHS, ITs, and TOs), and make recommendations to improve the use of health care services provided under the CHS program, including analyses of amounts reimbursed to providers, suppliers, and entities under CHS, compared to reimbursements through other public and private programs; barriers to access to health care under CHS; and adequacy of federal funding of CHS; and other matters that GAO determines appropriate.	9/23/2011
Sec. 201	Director of HIV/AIDS Prevention and Treatment	Requires the Director of the IHS office of HIV/AIDS Prevention and Treatment to submit a report to Congress describing the office's activities and findings related to HIV/AIDS prevention and treatment activities specific to Indians.	3/23/2012

Source: Prepared by the Congressional Research Service based on a review of the Patient Protection and Affordable Care Act ((PPACA) P.L. 111-148).

a. Sec. 801 requires the President to submit a report to Congress at the time that the budget is submitted. Per 31 U.S.C. § 1105(a) the President is required to submit his budget to Congress by the first Monday in February of the preceding fiscal year.

b. FY2011 budget was submitted prior to PPACA's enactment.

APPENDIX B. ACRONYMS USED IN THE REPORT

AG	Attorney General
BIA	Bureau of Indian Affairs
BIE	Bureau of Indian Education
CDC	Centers for Disease Control and Prevention
CHAP	Community Health Aide Program
CHEF	Catastrophic Health Emergency Fund
CHIP	Children's Health Insurance Program
CHS	Contract Health Services
CHSDA	Contract Health Services Delivery Area
CMS	Centers for Medicare and Medicaid Services
DOD	Department of Defense
FAD	Fetal Alcohol Disorder
FAS	Fetal Alcohol Spectrum
GAO	Government Accountability Office
HCERA	Health Care and Education Reconciliation Act
HHS	Department of Health and Human Services
HIPAA	Health Insurance Portability and Accountability Act
HIT	Health Information Technology
HUD	Department of Housing and Urban Development
IHCIA	Indian Health Care Improvement Act
IHCIF	Indian Health Care Improvement Fund
IHP	Indian Health Program
IHS	Indian Health Service
IRC	Internal Revenue Code
ISDEAA	Indian Self-Determination and Education Assistance Act
IT	Indian tribe
NHHCA	Native Hawaiian Health Care Act
NHSC	National Health Service Corp
PHS	Public Health Service
PHSA	Public Health Service Act
PPACA	Patient Protection and Affordable Care Act
SSA	Social Security Act
SAMSHA	Substance Abuse and Mental Health Services Administration
THP	Tribal Health Program
TO	tribal organization
UIHP	urban Indian health project
UIO	urban Indian organization
USC	U.S. Code
VA	Department of Veterans Affairs

End Notes

[1] P.L. 94-437, act of September 30, 1976, 90 Stat. 1400, as amended; 25 U.S.C. 1601 et seq., and 42 U.S.C. 1395qq, 1396j (and amending other sections).

[2] S. 1790 in the 111th Congress.

[3] See "Sec. 102. Findings" below.

[4] P.L. 102-573, act of October 29, 1992, 106 Stat. 4526. Previous reauthorizations occurred in 1980 (P.L. 96-537) and 1988 (P.L. 100-713), and substantial amendments were made in 1990 (P.L. 101-630, Title V).

[5] Omnibus Indian Advancement Act, P.L. 106-568, §815, act of December 27, 2000, 114 Stat. 2868, 2918.

[6] U.S. Department of Health and Human Services, Indian Health Service, IHS Fact Sheet: IHS Year 2010 Profile http://info.ihs.gov/Profile2010.asp.

[7] IHS provides services to American Indians and Alaska Natives residing in 35 states. Area offices may serve tribes in one state, such as the Alaska Area office that administers services in Alaska, or in multiple states, such as the Nashville area office that administers services for tribes on the east coast, in Alabama, Louisiana, and parts of Texas.

[8] Authorized by P.L. 93-638, the Indian Self-Determination and Education Assistance Act of January 4, 1975, 88 Stat. 2203, as amended; 25 U.S.C. 450 et seq.

[9] See "Sec. 102. Findings" below.

[10] Sec. 201(a), P.L. 81-152, act of June 30, 1949, 63 Stat. 377, 383, as amended; 40 U.S.C. 501.

[11] This program receives appropriations through the federal health center program. For more information, see http://bphc.hrsa.gov/about/specialpopulations.htm.

[12] P.L. 92-203, act of December 18, 1971, 85 Stat. 688, as amended; 43 U.S.C. 1601 et seq.

[13] P.L. 93-638, act of January 4, 1975, 88 Stat. 2203, as amended; 25 U.S.C. 450 et seq.

[14] 25 U.S.C. 47

[15] Title V of PPACA (Health Care Workforce) authorizes a number of new programs to augment the health care workforce and amends a number of existing programs. In a number of cases ITs, TOs, and UIOs may be eligible for these programs. See CRS Report R41278, *Public Health, Workforce, Quality, and Related Provisions in PPACA: Summary and Timeline*, coordinated by C. Stephen Redhead and Erin D. Williams.

[16] U.S. Department of Health and Human Services, Public Health Service, Indian Health Service, *Indian Health Service: Fiscal Year 2011 Justification of Estimates for Appropriations Committees* (Rockville, MD: HHS/PHS/IHS, 2009), pp. CJ-135; http://www.ihs.gov/Non Medical Programs/BudgetFormulation/documents/IHS%20FY%20201 1%20Congressional %20Justification.pdf.

[17] Ibid.

[18] The text below reflects the amendments that PPACA Sec. 1022 1(b)(1) made to this section.

[19] 28 U.S.C. 2415

[20] P.L. 104-191, act of August 21, 1996, 110 Stat. 1936, as amended.

[21] The text below reflects the amendments that PPACA Sec. 1022 1(b)(2) made to this section.

[22] The IHS FY2011 Justification of Estimates for Congressional Committees, available at http://www.ihs.gov/NonMedicalPrograms/BudgetFormulation/documents/IHS%20FY%202011%20Congressional%20Justification.pdf.

[23] The four types of facilities are inpatient health care facilities, outpatient health care facilities, staff quarters, and youth regional treatment centers.

[24] The specified workgroup and advisory board existed prior to enactment.

[25] IHCIA Section 801, which was not amended in PPACA, requires the President, each fiscal year to submit a number of required reports to Congress describing various IHCIA-authorized programs and other topics related to Indian health.

[26] IHS FY2011 Justification of Estimates for Congressional Committees, available at http://www.ihs.gov/NonMedicalPrograms/BudgetFormulation/documents/IHS%20FY%202011%20Congressional%20Justification.pdf.

[27] In order to be eligible for the CHS program, American Indians and Alaska Natives must be eligible for IHS services and live within a specified geographic area called a contract health service delivery area, or CHSDA.

[28] Section 508 of American Recovery and Reinvestment Act (P.L. 111-5) exempted American Indians and Alaska Natives from premiums and cost-sharing in Medicaid and CHIP. Sec. 2901 of PPACA also includes provisions to facilitate enrollment in Medicaid and CHIP. See description in CRS Report R41210, *Medicaid and the State Children's Health Insurance Program (CHIP) Provisions in PPACA: Summary and Timeline*, coordinated by Julie Stone.

[29] Under 5 U.S.C. Chapter 89.

[30] Under 5 U.S.C. Chapter 87.

[31] The Navajo reservation is located in parts of Arizona, Utah, and New Mexico.

[32] See U.S. Department of Health and Human Services, Indian Health Service, "Urban Indian Health Program: Program Overview." At http://www.ihs.gov/NonMedicalPrograms/Urban/Overview.asp.

[33] U.S. Department of Health and Human Services, Public Health Service, Indian Health Service, *Indian Health Service: Fiscal Year 2010 Justification of Estimates for Appropriations Committees* (Rockville, MD: HHS/PHS/IHS, 2009), p. CJ-133; http://www.ihs.gov/Non MedicalPrograms/BudgetFormulation/documents/ IHS_CJ_2010_Final_Submission.pdf.

[34] IHS is forbidden to bill or charge Indians (see 25 U.S.C. 1681 and 25 USC 458aaa-14), but IHCIA Title V does not prohibit UIHPs from charging their patients. "Sec. 197. Tribal Health Program Option for Cost Sharing" described below permits some THPs to charge for services.

[35] IHS, Office of Urban Indian Health Programs, *Urban Indian Health Program Statistics, FY2005* (Rockville, MD: October 16, 2007), p. 4.

[36] JCAHO now goes by the title The Joint Commission (TJC).

[37] See Title IV of P.L. 99-570.

[38] These locations are the Tanana Chiefs Conference, Incorporated and the Southeast Alaska Regional Health Corporation.

[39] The BIA's educational programs were transferred to a new agency, the Bureau of Indian Education (BIE), in 2006.

[40] P.L. 101-630, Title IV, act of November 28, 1990, 104 Stat. 4544, as amended; 25 U.S.C. 3202 et seq., 18 U.S.C. 1169.

[41] 5 U.S.C. 552.

[42] For more information about the National Health Service Corps, see CRS Report R40533, *Health Care Workforce: National Health Service Corps*, by Bernice Reyes-Akinbileje.

[43] Prior to the mark-up of the IHCIA Reauthorization and Extension Act by the Committee on Indian Affairs, the Act included provisions to amend the SSA. These provisions were either struck during the mark-up or were struck by Sec. 10221(b)(4).

[44] This program receives appropriations through the federal health center program. For more information, see http://bphc.hrsa.gov/about/specialpopulations.htm.

In: Indian Health Care ISBN: 978-1-61942-323-7
Editors J. Hansen and O. Bishop© 2012 Nova Science Publishers, Inc.

Chapter 3

INDIAN HEALTH SERVICE: INCREASED OVERSIGHT NEEDED TO ENSURE ACCURACY OF DATA USED FOR ESTIMATING CONTRACT HEALTH SERVICE NEED

United States Government Accountability Office

WHY GAO DID THIS STUDY

The Indian Health Service (IHS), an agency in the Department of Health and Human Services (HHS), provides health care to American Indians and Alaska Natives. When care at an IHS-funded facility is unavailable, IHS's contract health services (CHS) program pays for care from external providers if the patient meets certain requirements and funding is available. The Patient Protection and Affordable Care Act requires GAO to study the adequacy of federal funding for IHS's CHS program. To examine program funding needs, IHS collects data on unfunded services—services for which funding was not available—from the federal and tribal CHS programs. GAO examined (1) the extent to which IHS ensures the data it collects on unfunded services are accurate to determine a reliable estimate of CHS program need, (2) the extent to which federal and tribal CHS programs report having funds available to pay for contract health services, and (3) the experiences of external providers in obtaining payment from the CHS program. GAO surveyed 66 federal and 177 tribal CHS programs and spoke to IHS officials and 23 providers.

What GAO Recommends

GAO recommends that HHS direct IHS to ensure unfunded services data are accurately recorded, CHS program funds management is improved, and provider communication is enhanced. HHS noted how IHS would address the recommendations; describing the proposed new method to estimate need. IHS's steps will address some recommendations, but immediate steps are needed to improve the collection of unfunded services data to determine program need.

What GAO Found

Due to deficiencies in IHS's oversight of data collection, the data on unfunded services that IHS uses to estimate CHS program need were not accurate. Specifically, the data that IHS collected from CHS programs were incomplete and inconsistent. For example, 5 of the 66 federal and 30 of the 103 tribal CHS programs that responded to GAO's survey reported that they did not submit these data to IHS in fiscal year 2009. Also, the format of IHS's annual request has not provided the agency with complete information to determine which programs submitted these data. In addition, individual CHS programs reported inconsistencies in how they recorded information about a specific type of unfunded service that IHS uses in its assessment of need. A reliable estimate of need will require complete and consistent data from each of the individual CHS programs. In November 2010, IHS created a workgroup to examine weaknesses in its current data and explore other sources of data to estimate need. IHS officials expect the workgroup to make a recommendation to the IHS Director by the end of calendar year 2011 that IHS adopt a new method of estimating need. As of September 2011, IHS was continuing to develop this new method and officials indicated that deferral and denial data would continue to be collected until it makes further decisions about its needs assessment methodology.

Sixty of the 66 federal and 73 of the 103 tribal CHS programs that responded to GAO's survey reported that in fiscal year 2009 they did not have CHS funds available to pay for all services for which patients otherwise met requirements. Some federal CHS programs reported continuing to approve services for patients when sufficient funds were not available; IHS officials told us they were unaware this practice was occurring. In contrast, other federal CHS programs reported using a variety of strategies to help patients receive services outside of the CHS program in order to maximize the care that they could purchase. For example, some federal CHS programs reported helping patients locate free or low-cost health care. Tribal CHS programs reported using a variety of strategies not available to federal CHS programs. For example, 46 of 103 tribal CHS programs that responded to GAO's survey reported supplementing their CHS programs' funding with tribal funds, which are earned from tribal businesses or enterprises.

Most external providers that GAO interviewed described challenges in the CHS program payment process. For example, when patients presented for emergency services, 13 of 23 providers reported challenges determining which services would be approved for payment because, unlike other payers, they cannot check a patient's eligibility electronically. Eighteen providers noted challenges receiving communications from IHS about CHS policies and procedures related to payment, including having had few, if any, formal meetings with program staff and a lack of training and guidance. IHS officials acknowledged that the complexity of the CHS program makes provider education important. Most providers said that these challenges contributed to patient and provider burden. For example, providers said they generally billed the patient when CHS programs denied payment for services, although they rarely collected payment on care billed to CHS patients. Some providers said that this uncompensated care had not significantly affected them financially, but others stated that care uncompensated by the CHS program had affected them financially by, for example, limiting their ability to purchase new equipment.

ABBREVIATIONS

CHEF	Catastrophic Health Emergency Fund
CHS	contract health services
EMTALA	Emergency Medical Treatment and Active Labor Act
FDI	Federal Disparity Index
FEHBP	Federal Employees Health Benefits Program
HHS	Department of Health and Human Services
IHS	Indian Health Service
OIG	Office of Inspector General

September 23, 2011

Congressional Addressees

Access to health care services for American Indians and Alaska Natives has been a long-standing concern.[1] The Indian Health Service (IHS), an agency within the Department of Health and Human Services (HHS), is charged with providing health care to the approximately 1.9 million American Indians and Alaska Natives who are members or descendants of federally recognized tribes.[2] These services are provided at federally or tribally operated health care facilities,[3] which receive IHS funding and are located in 12 geographic regions overseen by IHS area offices.[4] These IHS-funded facilities vary in the services that they provide. For example, some facilities offer comprehensive hospital services, while others offer only primary care services. When services are not available at these facilities, the agency's contract health services (CHS) program may pay for services from external health care providers, including hospital- and office-based providers. The CHS program is administered at the local level by individual CHS programs generally affiliated with IHS-funded facilities in each area. These individual CHS programs may be federally or tribally operated.

These federal and tribal CHS programs determine whether or not to pay for the referral of a patient to an external provider or pay an external provider for a service already provided. IHS requires that patients meet certain eligibility and administrative requirements to have the services paid by the CHS program. In addition, the CHS program, which is funded through the annual appropriations process, must operate within the limits of its appropriations. Therefore, committees associated with each CHS program meet at least weekly to review cases and approve payment based on the relative medical need of each case. When the requirements have not been met or funds are not available, CHS programs defer or deny requests to pay for services. Services for which patients otherwise meet necessary requirements, but for which CHS program funds are not available for payment, are known as unfunded services.

Limits on available resources have affected the specific types of services available to American Indians and Alaska Natives through the CHS program. For example, in a 2005 report examining 13 IHS-funded health care facilities, we reported that primary care services were generally offered at the facilities, but certain specialty and other services were not always directly available to American Indians and Alaska Natives.[5] These facilities also generally lacked funds to pay for all of these services through their CHS programs. We also noted that, in some cases, gaps in services resulted in diagnosis or treatment delays that exacerbated the severity of a patient's condition and required more intensive treatment.

Funding for the CHS program has increased significantly, from $498 million in fiscal year 2005 to $779 million in fiscal year 2010. Despite the funding increases over this period, IHS reported an increase in the number of services denied by CHS programs due to a lack of funding. IHS uses the number of services that were deferred or denied due to a lack of funds by the CHS programs to develop an estimate of the additional funds needed for the CHS program. However, IHS and other stakeholders have questioned whether these data on unfunded services represent the extent of need. For example, IHS has acknowledged that little is known about the extent of unfunded services for tribal CHS programs. Just for federal CHS programs, IHS has estimated that $360 million in services were unfunded in fiscal year 2008.[6]

The Patient Protection and Affordable Care Act requires GAO to study the adequacy of federal funding for the CHS program.[7] IHS does not maintain comprehensive data and information about the program that would be relevant to assessing the adequacy of federal funding. As discussed with the committees of jurisdiction, we examine (1) the extent to which IHS ensures the data it collects on unfunded services are accurate to determine a reliable estimate of CHS program need, (2) the extent to which federal and tribal CHS programs report having funds available to pay for contract health services, and (3) the experiences of external providers in obtaining payment from the CHS program.

To examine the extent to which IHS ensures the data it collects on unfunded services are accurate to determine a reliable estimate of CHS program need and the extent to which federal and tribal CHS programs report having funds available to pay for contract health services, we administered a Web-based survey to the 66 federal CHS programs identified by the area offices. We administered the survey between October 2010 and January 2011 and received completed survey responses from all 66 federal CHS programs. We also administered a mixed-mode survey—both Web-based and by mail—to the 177 tribal CHS programs identified by the area offices. We administered the survey between September 2010 and January 2011 and received completed survey responses from 103 of the tribal CHS programs, for a response rate of 58 percent. Because we did not receive responses from all tribal CHS programs and because there is variability among programs due to the flexibility tribes and tribal organizations have in administering their programs, the results from our survey of tribal CHS programs are not generalizable to all tribal CHS programs. In addition, we conducted two site visits to IHS's

Oklahoma City and Portland area offices, interviewed officials from IHS and each of IHS's 12 area offices to discuss oversight of the CHS program, and spoke with tribal health advocacy groups. We also examined IHS oversight—such as the provision of policy and guidance—conducted to ensure that CHS programs consistently and completely record and report unfunded services data. We compared these oversight activities to the standards described in the *Standards for Internal Control in the Federal Government* and the *Internal Control Management and Evaluation Tool.*[8] We also reviewed our cost estimating guide to assess procedures for determining a reliable estimate for budgetary purposes.[9]

To examine the experiences of external providers in obtaining payment from the CHS program, we interviewed representatives from hospitals and office-based health care providers in selected IHS areas. We selected four areas based on their per capita CHS funding for fiscal year 2009 and dependency on CHS funds for hospital services.[10] The four areas we selected were Bemidji, Billings, Phoenix, and Oklahoma City,[11] which represent areas that were above or below average for each of our selection criteria. Within these four areas, we selected 16 hospitals and 7 office-based providers from a list of providers that were identified by federal CHS programs in our survey and by other experts as interacting frequently with IHS's CHS program. Given the small number of providers in our sample and our process for selecting them, the results from these interviews are not generalizable to all providers interacting with the CHS program. We asked providers about their experiences obtaining effective and timely communication related to the payment process, such as training or guidance on determining patient eligibility for CHS program payment of services, and determining the status of claims or receiving payment, and compared their experiences with the standards described in the *Standards for Internal Control in the Federal Government* and the *Internal Control Management and Evaluation Tool.*[12] We asked providers a standard set of open-ended questions and we did not independently validate their reported experiences, but we did discuss many of the issues they raised with IHS officials. (See app. I for more details on our scope and methodology.)

We conducted this performance audit from January 2010 to September 2011 in accordance with generally accepted government auditing standards. Those standards require that we plan and perform the audit to obtain sufficient, appropriate evidence to provide a reasonable basis for our findings and conclusions based on our audit objectives. We believe that the evidence obtained provides a reasonable basis for our findings and conclusions based on our audit objectives.

Background

IHS oversees the CHS program through 12 area offices. Federal and tribal CHS programs in each of these areas pay for services from external providers if services are not available directly through IHS-funded facilities, if patients meet certain requirements, and if funds are available. IHS conducts an annual assessment to estimate CHS program need. To perform its needs assessment, IHS requests data from area offices and individual CHS programs on health care services they were unable to fund.

CHS Program Organization

IHS manages the CHS program through a decentralized system of 12 area offices, which oversee individual CHS programs in 35 states where many American Indian and Alaska Native communities are located. (See figure 1 for a map of the counties included in the 12 areas. Residence in these counties is generally a requirement for obtaining contract health services.)

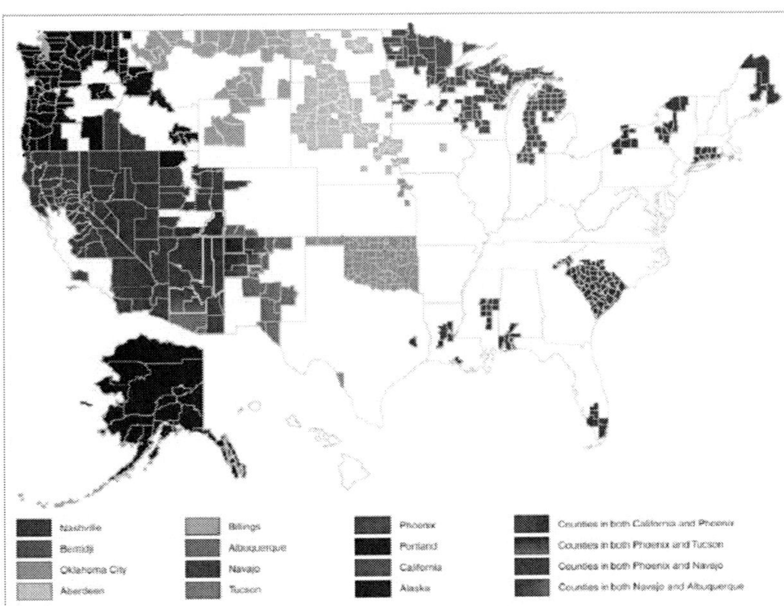

Source: GAO analysis of IHS information, as of July 2011.

Figure 1. Counties in the 12 IHS Areas.

IHS headquarters is responsible for overseeing the CHS program. Among other things, it sets program policy and distributes CHS program funds to the 12 area offices. The 12 area offices then distribute funds to CHS programs within their respective areas, monitor the CHS programs, establish procedures within the policies set by IHS, and provide programs with guidance and technical assistance. About 46 percent of CHS funds are distributed to federal CHS programs and the other 54 percent to tribal CHS programs.[13] Tribal CHS programs must meet the same statutory and regulatory requirements as federal CHS programs, but they are not generally subject to the same policies, procedures, and reporting requirements established for federal CHS programs.[14]

Federal and tribal CHS programs pay for services from external providers if the services are not available at IHS-funded facilities. The services purchased include hospital, specialty physician, outpatient, laboratory, dental, radiology, pharmacy, and transportation services. While programs may have agreements or contracts with providers, they are not required for a provider to be paid. For example, a CHS program may have a contract with a nearby hospital or specialty providers, such as an orthopedic practice, to provide services to American Indians and Alaska Natives served by the CHS program. However, in the event of an emergency, patients have the option of visiting the nearest available provider, regardless of whether that provider has any prior relationship with the CHS program.

Patients must meet certain eligibility, administrative, and medical priority requirements to have their services paid for by the CHS program. (See table 1.) To be eligible to receive services through the CHS program, patients must be members of federally recognized tribes and live in specific areas. In addition, patients must meet specific administrative requirements. For example, if there are other health care resources available to a patient, such as Medicaid and Medicare,[15] these resources must pay for services before the CHS program because the CHS program is generally the payer of last resort.[16] If a patient has met these requirements, a program committee (often including medical staff) that is part of the local CHS program evaluates the medical necessity of the service. IHS has established four broad medical priority levels of health care services eligible for payment and a fifth for excluded services that cannot be paid for with CHS program funds. Each area office is required to establish priorities that are consistent with these medical priority levels and are adapted to the specific needs of the CHS programs in their area. Federal CHS programs must assign a priority level to services based on the priority system established by their area office. Funds permitting, federal CHS programs first pay for the highest priority services (priority level I: emergent/acutely urgent care), and then for all or only some of the lower priority services they fund. Tribal CHS programs must use medical priorities when making funding decisions, but unlike federal CHS programs, they may develop a system that differs from the set of priorities established by IHS.

There are two primary paths through which patients may have their care paid for by a federal CHS program. The subsequent sections generally describe these two paths, which IHS officials told us federal CHS programs are expected to follow. First, a patient may obtain a referral from a provider at an IHS-funded health care facility to receive services from an external provider, such as a hospital or office-based physician. That referral is submitted to the CHS program for review. If the patient meets the requirements and the CHS program has funding available, the services in the referral are approved by the CHS program and a purchase order is issued to the external provider and sent to IHS's fiscal intermediary.[17] Once the patient receives the services from the external provider, that provider obtains payment for the services in the approved referral by sending a claim to IHS's fiscal intermediary. Second, in the case of an emergency, the patient may seek care from an external provider without first obtaining a referral. Once that care is provided, the external provider must send the patient's medical records and a claim for payment to the CHS program.[18] At that time, the CHS program will determine if the patient meets the necessary program requirements and CHS funding is available for a purchase order to be issued and sent to the fiscal intermediary. As in the earlier instance, the provider obtains payment by submitting a claim to IHS's fiscal intermediary. Patients seeking to have their care paid for by tribal CHS programs follow similar pathways, but these programs have certain flexibilities. For example, while some tribal CHS programs also contract with IHS's fiscal intermediary to pay claims, they may also utilize other arrangements. (See figure 2 for an overview of these two paths for a patient to access the CHS program.)

Within either of these pathways, if the CHS program determines that the patient's service does not meet the necessary requirements or funding is not available, it denies CHS funding. It may also defer funding a service. The CHS program may issue a deferral when CHS funds are not available for a service but the patient has otherwise met the eligibility and administrative requirements.[19]

Table 1. Requirements for Approving Care for CHS Funding

Category	Requirement[a,b]
Eligibility	• Individual is a member or descendant of a federally recognized tribe or maintains close social and economic ties with the tribe. • Individual lives on a federally recognized Indian reservation or within the designated service delivery area for the CHS program.
Administrative	• Any available alternate source of payment for care, such as Medicare, Medicaid, or private insurance, for which an individual is eligible, must be used before the CHS program will pay. • IHS-funded facility is not reasonably available and accessible to provide the care. • Prior approval is obtained for non-emergency services. • For emergency services, the CHS program is notified within 72 hours of the care being provided or within 30 days for elderly and disabled persons.
Medical Priority	Each area office is required to establish priorities that are consistent with IHS's medical priority levels and that are adapted to the specific needs of the CHS programs in their area. In contrast, tribes have flexibility to create their own priorities, which can differ from IHS's. Below are the medical priority levels established by IHS.[c] • Priority level I, includes emergent/acutely urgent care services, such as trauma care, acute/chronic renal replacement therapy, obstetrical delivery and neonatal care. Priority level II, includes preventive care services, such as preventive ambulatory care, routine prenatal care, and screening mammograms. • Priority level III, includes primary and secondary care services, such as scheduled ambulatory services for nonemergent conditions, elective surgeries, and specialty consultations. • Priority level IV, includes chronic tertiary and extended care services, such as rehabilitation care, skilled nursing facility care, and organ transplants. • Priority level V, includes excluded services, such as cosmetic plastic surgery and experimental procedures, that programs may not pay for with CHS program funds.

Source: GAO analysis of IHS's Indian Health Manual and regulations, which can be found at 42 C.F.R. §§ 136.23, 136.61 (2010).

[a] If eligibility, administrative, and medical priority requirements have been met, but funds are not available, care is to be deferred or denied.

[b] There are also certain exceptions to these requirements.

[c] Funds permitting, federal CHS programs first pay for all of the highest priority services, and then all or some of the lower priority services, but CHS program funds may not be used to pay for priority level V services.

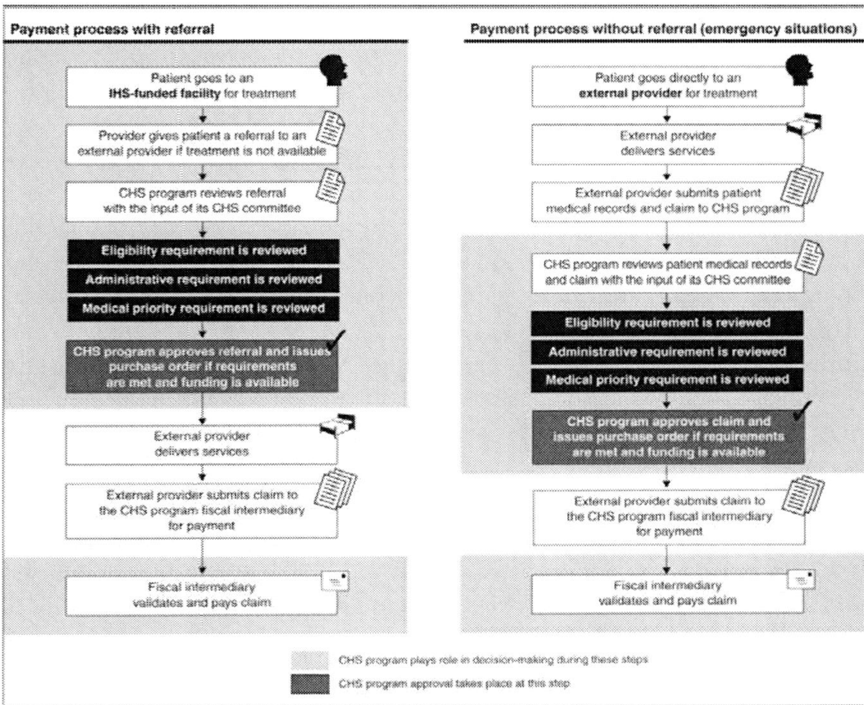

Figure 2. Two Paths for Patient Care to Be Funded by a Federal CHS Program.

Needs Assessment for the CHS Program

IHS conducts an annual assessment to estimate the CHS program's unmet need, which helps inform its budget request for the CHS program. To gather information for its needs assessment, IHS headquarters sends an annual request for information to each of the 12 area offices asking them to report information from the federal and tribal CHS programs in their respective areas. The annual request contains a template that asks each area office to provide, among other things, summary counts of deferrals and denials that were recorded by the CHS programs in their areas. For example, each area office is asked to provide areawide totals of the number of new deferrals that remained unfunded at the end of the fiscal year. They are also to provide summary counts of denials that have been issued for each of eight categories of denial reasons, regardless of the type of service denied. The eight categories generally correspond to the CHS program's eligibility, administrative, and medical priority requirements.[20] Although funding for a service may be denied for multiple reasons, programs are required to categorize each denial by a single primary reason.

IHS uses the data recorded by the individual CHS programs and collected by the area offices to develop an estimate of the CHS program's unmet need. (See figure 3.) To develop its estimate, IHS headquarters adds the total number of reported deferrals and the total number of denials reported in one of eight IHS-defined denial categories: "care not within medical priority." According to IHS, CHS programs are only to record a denial as "care not within medical priority" to indicate that the patient met eligibility and administrative requirements, but the care requested was not within one of the medical priority levels for which funding was available. For example, a program that determines it only has funding available to pay for care designated as priority level I may deny a request to pay for care designated as priority level II because the care requested was not within the medical priority for which funding was available. Although IHS requests that the area offices report data from both federal and tribal CHS programs, it cannot require tribal CHS programs to report these data. Therefore, IHS officials told us they make an assumption in their assessment of program need that most tribal CHS programs do not report deferral and denial counts to the area offices. Because tribal programs receive about half of IHS's CHS funding, and because IHS believes that tribal CHS programs' experiences are similar to federal programs, IHS takes the data reported by area offices and multiplies them by two to calculate an estimate of the total number of deferrals and denials for the entire CHS program. IHS then multiplies this count of deferrals and denials by an estimated average cost per claim (calculated using a weighted average of the costs for inpatient and outpatient paid CHS claims) to develop an estimate of the funds needed for the CHS program. To this estimate, IHS adds data from the CHS program's Catastrophic Health Emergency Fund (CHEF), a fund that IHS headquarters administers to reimburse CHS programs for their expenses from high-cost medical cases.[21] Specifically, IHS adds the total billed charges from services for which CHS programs sought reimbursement from IHS headquarters through CHEF, but that CHEF was unable to fund. (See app. II for further discussion of CHEF.)

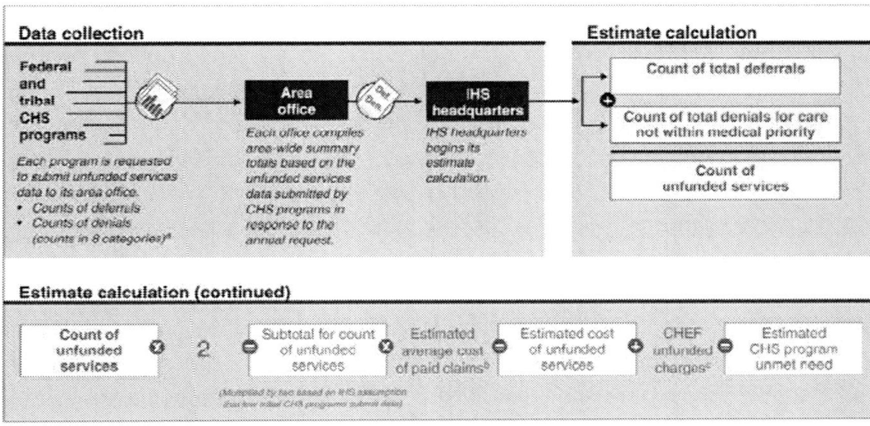

Source: GAO interviews with IHS officials and analysis of IHS documents.

[a] The eight categories of denial are: (1) eligible but care not within medical priority, (2) eligible but alternate resource available, (3) patient ineligible for CHS, (4) emergency notification not within 72 hours, (5) non-emergency prior approval not authorized, (6) patient resides outside CHS delivery area, (7) IHS facility available and accessible, and (8) all other denials.

[b] IHS estimates an average cost per claim by calculating a weighted average of the costs for inpatient and outpatient paid CHS claims. IHS then multiplies this estimate by the count of deferrals and denials.

[c] The Catastrophic Health Emergency Fund (CHEF) is administered by IHS headquarters to reimburse CHS programs for their expenses from high cost medical cases. IHS adds the total billed charges from services for which CHS programs sought reimbursement from IHS headquarters through CHEF, but that CHEF was unable to fund.

Figure 3. IHS Process for Collecting Unfunded Services Data and Estimating the CHS Program's Unmet Need.

IHS's Oversight of Data Collection Does Not Ensure the Accuracy of the Data Used for Estimating CHS Program Need

Due to deficiencies in IHS's oversight of data collection, the unfunded services data on deferrals and denials that IHS used to estimate program need are incomplete and inconsistent. IHS does not have complete deferral and denial data from all federal and tribal CHS programs to estimate CHS program need. While IHS headquarters told us that area offices submit a report on unfunded services from their federal and tribal CHS programs in response to the annual request,[22] these reports did not include data from all federal or tribal CHS programs. Of the 66 federal CHS programs that responded to our survey, 5 reported that they did not submit any deferral or denial data to their area offices in response to IHS's annual request in fiscal year 2009. IHS officials acknowledged that they did not follow up with federal CHS programs to ensure they submitted data. Although not required, tribal programs may choose to submit deferral and denial data to IHS and the agency asks the area offices to include tribal data in their annual reports. Of the 103 tribal CHS programs that responded to our survey, 30 indicated that they collected data on unfunded services and submitted these data to their area offices in response to IHS's annual request in fiscal year 2009.[23] IHS officials acknowledged that the agency needed to provide more outreach and technical assistance to tribal programs to submit data in response to IHS's annual request. For example, they told us that an area office used such efforts during one fiscal year and was successful at eliciting data submissions from more tribes. By not encouraging the reporting of unfunded services data from all programs, IHS's data collection activities are not consistent with the *Standards for Internal Control in the Federal Government*, which state that an organization's management should provide reasonable assurance of the reliability of its reporting data for the agency to achieve its goals—in this instance, IHS's goal to appropriately determine CHS program need. As we have also previously reported, the ability to generate reliable estimates is a critical function for agency management; having accurate data contributes to the reliability of the estimate.[24]

Second, IHS's report template was not designed to allow the agency to collect complete information for estimating need because it did not distinguish between the federal and tribal CHS programs that did report data. Because IHS headquarters only requested areawide totals in its report template, IHS officials were unable to determine which CHS programs reported data from the area reports that were submitted. IHS officials told us they did not know how many federal or tribal CHS programs reported data, although they estimated that most of the data were from federal programs and only a small percentage were from tribal programs. To account for the lack of complete data from tribal programs, when conducting its needs assessment, IHS doubled the count of unfunded services it received from the area offices. However, this means that any data received from tribal programs were being doubled along with the federal data, contributing to an unreliable estimate of need. For example, in fiscal year 2009, one area office reported a total of 4,858 denials for "care not within medical priority," which IHS doubled to account for the lack of complete data from tribal programs. However, we determined that 2,901 of the 4,858 denials were reported by tribal CHS programs.[25] IHS officials told us that they do not distinguish federal and tribal CHS program data in their annual data reporting template because they believe the data they receive from tribal CHS programs are so limited that they would not significantly affect their estimate of need.

Additionally, CHS programs inconsistently categorized a specific type of denial reason that is reported to IHS headquarters and used in its estimate of CHS program need because IHS has not provided guidance on this issue. CHS programs can deny care for multiple reasons, but IHS requires CHS programs to select a primary reason for denial. Specifically, IHS officials told us that IHS only counted those denials with a primary reason identified as "care not within medical priority" in its needs assessment because these services were denied solely if funds were not available.[26] However, neither IHS headquarters nor the area offices had provided guidance to federal CHS programs on how to select this primary reason for denial. Consequently, we found some area office and CHS program officials defined this type of denial reason in different ways. Officials from four area offices told us that they defined denials for "care not within medical priority" as also including services denied for administrative reasons or services that are excluded even if CHS funds are available such as cosmetic or experimental procedures. In our survey of the 66 federal CHS programs, 51 reported that they would apply this denial category if the care requested was an excluded service. One CHS program reported not knowing that a primary reason for denial existed. Because this category of denial was the only denial reason IHS used in its estimate, inconsistencies in how this denial reason was categorized by CHS programs have directly affected IHS's estimate of need.

Some CHS programs also inconsistently recorded deferrals because IHS has not provided guidance about how it uses deferral data in its needs assessment. IHS officials told us that both deferral and denial data were used in IHS's needs assessment. However, officials from one area office reported that their understanding was that only denials were counted in IHS's needs assessment. In our survey of the 66 federal CHS programs, we found that 15 reported recording a decision to defer a service as both a deferral and a denial (making the count of denials inaccurate). Because IHS uses both deferrals and denials to estimate need, the inconsistent recording of deferrals would directly affect IHS's estimate of need. IHS did not have a written policy documenting how the deferral and denial data it requests annually from the CHS programs would be used in its needs assessment and IHS officials told us they had not provided training to area offices or CHS programs on how to complete the annual request.[27] However, this lack of guidance is inconsistent with the *Standards for Internal Control in the Federal Government*, which notes that formally documented policies and procedures provide guidance that, among other things, helps to ensure that staff perform activities consistently across an agency.[28]

IHS officials have also identified weaknesses in the deferral and denial data that they used to estimate CHS program need. For example, they told us the data did not capture complete information on needed services that were not requested of the CHS programs because patients may have been discouraged from presenting for care or providers may have chosen not to write referrals if they believed funds were not available to pay for services.[29] IHS officials also told us that these data did not capture data on the extent to which tribes supplemented their CHS funds with tribal funds to avoid deferring or denying health care services.[30]

IHS has initiated steps to examine these weaknesses in its current data and explore other sources of data to estimate CHS program need. In November 2010, IHS convened an Unmet Needs Data Subcommittee as part of its Director's Workgroup on Improving the CHS Program.[31] The subcommittee was comprised of representatives from federal and tribal CHS programs. In a January 2011 report, the subcommittee noted that IHS's deferral and denial data had inaccuracies. While the report noted that reliably captured deferral and denial data on all patients would present the strongest evidence of need, it acknowledged that these data were incompletely and inconsistently reported by CHS programs, and recognized that this undermined the reliability of the estimated need IHS reports to the Committees on Appropriations annually in its budget justification. In February 2011, the subcommittee presented options for improving IHS's assessment of CHS program need to the Director's Workgroup.

Based on these options, the Director's Workgroup agreed that the subcommittee should explore a new methodology for estimating CHS program funding needs that relies on different sources of data. Rather than relying on deferral and denial data, the new method would use IHS's existing Federal Disparity Index (FDI). IHS calculates the FDI to estimate the disparity between its overall health care funding and the amount of funding needed to provide care to American Indians and Alaska Natives at a level comparable to the care provided by the Federal Employees Health Benefits Program (FEHBP), which is a nationwide health insurance program available to federal employees.[32] With this new method, IHS would adapt the FDI to calculate an estimate of need for each CHS program. Specifically, each IHS-funded facility would use a standardized tool to (1) calculate what proportion of services is paid for by its CHS program because these services are not available on-site at an IHS-funded facility, (2) estimate the level of CHS funding that would be needed to provide comparable services to those covered by FEHBP, and (3) compare that estimated level of funding to the program's actual level of funding. As a first step, each IHS area was to pilot the methodology on- site at two of its IHS-funded facilities. Once the pilots were completed, IHS officials told us the Workgroup planned to review the results of these pilots and issue a final report that contains a recommendation for the Director of IHS to consider for approval. As of September 2011, IHS officials said that they had finished the on-site pilots, but they were still making decisions about how to best adapt the FDI method to estimate CHS program need and they did not have a formal agency approved plan for implementing it. Officials indicated that they expected the Workgroup to issue a final report to the Director for approval by the end of calendar year 2011.

In addition to the proposed new method for estimating need, the Director's Workgroup agreed that actions be taken to improve the agency's collection of deferral and denial data that is currently used for that purpose. However, as of September 2011, IHS officials told us that the agency had not determined whether it would make improvements to the collection of deferral and denial data because it had not determined how such data would be used if the FDI method is adopted. But, officials said that they still see merit in using deferral and denial data to estimate CHS program need and, therefore, IHS may supplement the estimates from the FDI method with deferral and denial data from CHS programs that agency officials believe collect accurate data. IHS officials indicated that, until this decision is made, the agency will continue to collect deferral and denial data from the area offices through its annual request.

Most Federal and Tribal CHS Programs Reported They Did Not Have CHS Funds Available to Pay for All Services

Most federal and tribal CHS programs reported that they did not have CHS funds available to pay for all services for patients who otherwise met eligibility and administrative requirements in fiscal year 2009. In addition, some federal CHS programs reported using problematic funds management practices.

Most Federal CHS Programs Reported That They Did Not Have CHS Funds Available to Pay for All Services, and Some Reported Using Problematic Funds Management Practices

Of the 66 federal CHS programs that responded to our survey, 60 reported that they did not have CHS funds available to pay for all services for patients who otherwise met eligibility and administrative requirements in fiscal year 2009.[33] IHS officials told us that most CHS programs establish budgets as a way to help ensure that funds are available throughout the year.[34] However, even with this budgeting, 11 of these 60 CHS programs reported that they depleted their funds before the end of the fiscal year. Officials from three CHS programs we spoke with said their programs experienced multiple high-cost cases in the fourth quarter that depleted their funds. An official from another CHS program noted that the program is located in a rural area and the closest specialty care providers are 3 hours away by car. Therefore, if emergency care is required, the patient must be transported by air, which the CHS official said is expensive. In our survey, each federal CHS program identified the three most common categories of services it deferred or denied in fiscal year 2009. The most commonly cited categories of services were dental services, orthopedic services, vision services, and diagnostic and imaging services.[35]

The 60 federal CHS programs that reported not having CHS funds available to pay for all services in fiscal year 2009 varied in the extent to which they had funds available to pay for services in each of the priority levels. Some programs described the circumstances that influenced the extent to which they had funds available to pay for services in fiscal year 2009. (See figure 4.)

- Thirty-nine of these programs reported having funds available to pay for all priority level I services (emergent/acutely urgent care) and some services in lower priority levels. Some of these CHS programs said that after purchasing all of their priority level I services, they had funds remaining at the end of the fiscal year and were able to use these funds to pay for lower priority services for patients whose services they had originally deferred or denied. For example, officials from one CHS program reported that in fiscal year 2009, they were able to use funds at the end of the fiscal year to provide eyeglasses to children and the elderly; a lower priority service that normally would not have been funded.
- Ten of these programs reported having funds available to pay for all priority level I services, but no services in lower priority levels. Some of these CHS programs reported that they never fund services beyond priority level I because their funds are so limited. An official from one of these programs noted that if a patient's case was originally deferred or denied because it was not a priority level I service but the patient's condition became more severe, the case may later be reclassified as a priority level I and the services purchased.
- Six of these programs reported having funds available to pay for some of their priority level I services and some services in lower priority levels. An official from one of these CHS programs told us that they strictly adhere to a weekly budget. For example, if they approved three high-cost cancer treatment cases one week, they may deny other priority level I cases because they do not have funds remaining to pay for these services. But, if funds in another week are sufficient to pay for all priority level I cases, they may also have funds available to pay for some lower priority services. An official from another of these CHS programs told us that staffing shortages over 2 years resulted in the program paying for services as the requests were received rather than funding them in order of medical priority. The official told us that, as a result, the CHS program paid for some priority level IV services, like durable medical equipment, even though they did not have funds available to pay for all of their priority level I services for the year.
- Five of these programs reported depleting their CHS funds before the end of the fiscal year and reported that they did not have funds available to pay for all priority level I services. One of these programs reported depleting its funds for the fiscal year in the second quarter of

fiscal year 2009, two programs reported depleting their funds in the third quarter, and two programs reported depleting their funds in the fourth quarter.

Federal CHS programs we spoke with reported using a variety of strategies to help patients receive services outside of the CHS program in order to maximize the care that they could purchase. For example, strategies noted by some CHS programs included helping patients locate free or low-cost health care or negotiating reduced rates with providers on the patient's behalf. Although CHS programs are required to identify alternate resources before approving a referral, some officials we spoke with said they have implemented additional measures to help enroll patients in alternate coverage, such as Medicare and Medicaid. For example, one CHS program reported hiring a benefits coordinator who is responsible for helping enroll people in alternate coverage.

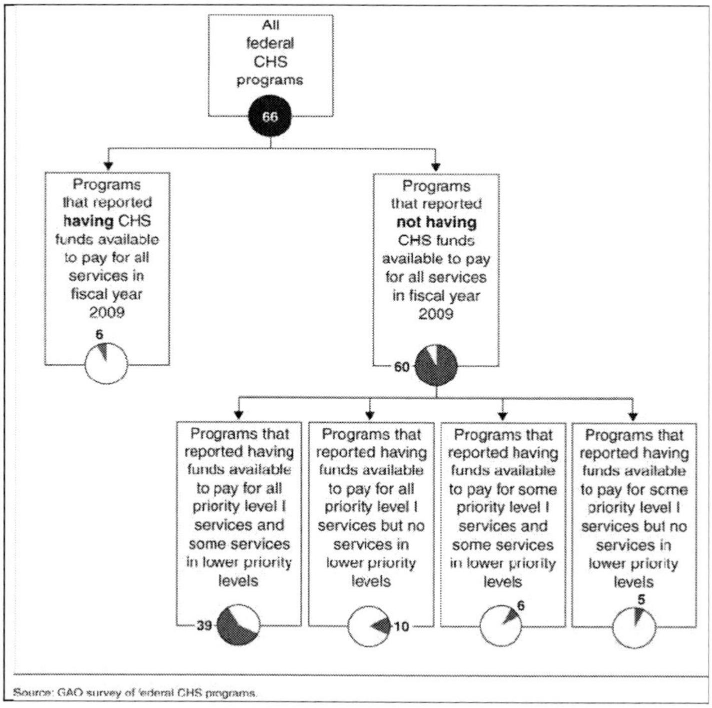

Figure 4. Priority Levels for Which Federal CHS Programs Had Funds Available to Pay for Services in Fiscal Year 2009.

IHS's CHS programs are not able to pay for services for all patients who meet program requirements because they must operate within the limited funding available. Whenever a program incurs costs for services, the program incurs legal obligations to make payments. IHS does not authorize programs to incur obligations in excess of their "allowances," which are distributions of funds that IHS makes to programs from appropriations for contract health services.[36,37] According to IHS officials, programs are expected to actively manage their funds in order to maximize the care that can be purchased, and defer or deny care when sufficient funds are not available. Officials from five federal CHS programs told us, however, that they approved services when funds were depleted for a fiscal year with the understanding that providers would not be paid until the next fiscal year. For example, one of these officials reported that at the beginning of fiscal year 2009, the program owed $2 million to providers for care provided in fiscal year 2008 for which funds had not been available. At least one of these officials believed that she was not authorized to deny care due to lack of funds.

The reports from these officials suggest significant weaknesses in funds management and violations of IHS policy creating the potential for violations of the Antideficiency Act.[38] They also suggest significant inconsistencies in the administration of federal CHS programs. When asked about this issue, IHS officials told us that they were not aware that CHS programs had approved services without available funds, but acknowledged that there had been some confusion in the past regarding programs' authority to deny care when funds were not available. They also noted that the agency guidance on funds management that is provided to CHS program staff is vague and needs to be updated and clarified. The officials told us that the agency plans to update and revise relevant IHS guidance, but had not developed a timeline for these revisions. The officials said that they have delegated responsibility to the area offices for issuing specific guidance to CHS programs, as well as conducting oversight regarding funds management and other issues. The officials, however, acknowledged that additional guidance and training from IHS headquarters for the CHS programs on funds management would be helpful.

Most Tribal CHS Programs Reported That They Did Not Have CHS Funds Available to Pay for All Services but Many Used other Strategies to Expand Access to Care

Of the 103 tribal CHS programs that responded to our survey, most reported they did not have CHS funds available to pay for all services for patients who otherwise met eligibility and administrative requirements, with 73 reporting that they depleted their CHS funds at some point during fiscal year 2009.[39] In our survey, each tribal CHS program identified the three most common categories of services that were requested but not funded in fiscal year 2009. The most commonly cited categories of services that were requested but not funded were dental services, orthopedic services, prescription drugs, diagnostic and imaging services, and hospital services.[40]

Tribal CHS programs reported using a variety of strategies not available to federal CHS programs to expand access to care. Forty-six of the 103 tribal CHS programs that responded to our survey reported supplementing their CHS programs' funding with tribal funds—funds earned from tribal businesses or enterprises.[41] For example, one tribal CHS program we spoke with used the profits from its tribally funded medical and dental clinics, which served non-IHS patients on a fee-forservice basis, to supplement its CHS funding. Of the 46 programs that reported finding it necessary to supplement their CHS programs with tribal funds, 28 reported contributing as much as was needed each year, while the other 18 reported that their tribal contributions were limited by the availability of funds from year to year. In our survey, tribal CHS programs identified the three most common categories of services paid for with tribal funds in fiscal year 2009. The most commonly cited categories of services were prescription drugs, dental services, hospital services, and orthopedic services. Five tribal CHS programs we spoke with reported using tribal funds to expand access to contract health services to individuals living outside the designated CHS delivery area, or to pay for services CHS funding would not usually cover.

Tribal CHS programs also reported supplementing their CHS funding by using reimbursements from third party payers to pay for CHS services, a strategy not available to federal CHS programs. Thirty-four of the 103 tribal CHS programs that responded to our survey reported using reimbursements for services provided at their IHS-funded facilities from third party payers such as Medicare, Medicaid, or private insurance to pay for additional services through their CHS programs. One tribal CHS program we spoke with reported that more than half of its budget relied on funds from third party reimbursements, although officials noted that even with this supplemental funding, they were still limited to funding priority level I services only.

In addition, five tribal CHS programs we spoke with reported using strategies to expand access to care that reduced their reliance on CHS funds. For example, two programs we spoke with were able to directly enroll patients in a state-based insurance program for low-income individuals who did not qualify for Medicaid, and to pay the premiums using tribal funds. For uninsured CHS-eligible patients who are ineligible for government programs, one program reported using its IHS-allocated CHS funds to purchase private insurance coverage under a waiver from IHS.[42] Enrolling eligible patients in alternate coverage reduced the reliance on CHS funds because the CHS program would only have to pay for services to the extent they are not covered by the alternate resources. Another program was able to achieve cost savings by contracting with a third party administrator to process its CHS claims, which allowed it to access a preferred provider network that provided care at discounted rates. Officials from another program reported bringing specialty providers, such as cardiologists and ear, nose, and throat specialists on- site at their facility to save money, compared to what it would cost to pay providers in the community for individual services.

MOST EXTERNAL PROVIDERS REPORTED CHALLENGES WITH THE CHS PROGRAM PAYMENT PROCESS THAT MAY BURDEN BOTH PATIENTS AND PROVIDERS

Most of the external providers who we interviewed reported challenges in determining patient eligibility for CHS payment of services, in obtaining CHS payment, and in receiving communications on CHS policies and procedures from IHS related to payment. Providers stated that these challenges contributed to patient and provider burdens.

Most Providers Reported Challenges Determining Patient Eligibility, in Obtaining Payment, and in Receiving Communications on CHS Policies and Procedures Related to Payment

Thirteen of the 23 providers who we interviewed reported challenges in determining whether patients presenting for care without a CHS referral were eligible to have services paid by the CHS program. Fourteen providers also reported challenges obtaining timely payment from CHS programs. Lastly, 18 providers noted challenges receiving communications from IHS about CHS policies and procedures related to payment, including having had few, if any, formal meetings with CHS staff and a lack of training and guidance.

Determining Patient Eligibility for CHS Program Payment of Services

Thirteen providers who we interviewed reported challenges determining whether patient services would be approved by the CHS program for payment. Providers interact with American Indian and Alaska Native patients if these patients bring a referral from an IHS-funded health care facility. In the case of an emergency, a patient may seek care without obtaining a prior referral. Thirteen providers said it was especially challenging to determine patient eligibility when patients presented for care without a CHS program referral. Six providers noted that for other payers with which they interact, they are able to electronically check a patient's eligibility or covered services. However, IHS officials indicated that it is not possible for providers to check electronically whether the CHS program will pay for a service. Five providers indicated that, when possible, they attempted to contact the CHS programs in order to obtain information about a patient's eligibility. However, those providers said they were generally not able to get in contact with CHS program staff. Moreover, even if a provider determined that a patient met some CHS program eligibility requirements, such as tribal membership, payment was still conditional on whether the CHS program reviewed the patient's medical record and later determined that the emergency service met medical priority requirements and funds were available. Therefore, providers may not know if they will receive payment for services delivered to the patient until the claim they have submitted to the CHS program is reviewed. In the absence of a process to determine patient eligibility for the CHS program, 12 providers said they submit claims for payment to CHS programs for all patients who self-identified as being American Indian or Alaska Native or eligible for the CHS program.

Fourteen providers said that when a patient presented for care with a CHS program referral, the likelihood that they would receive payment for the services delivered to the patient increased. For example, one provider stated that for the care delivered to American Indian and Alaska Native patients without a CHS program referral, about 80 percent of claims were denied; in comparison, about 20 percent of claims were denied when patients had a CHS referral. IHS officials said that denials may occur for a patient who has a referral if the patient presented for care at the external provider before the referral was approved by the CHS program committee.[43] However, they also noted that there were situations in which a referral that had been approved by a CHS program committee could still be denied. For example, if a patient did not apply for alternate resources, such as Medicare and Medicaid, for which the patient was eligible or the provider did not bill other payers for which the patient was eligible, the claim may be denied for CHS payment.[44] Additionally, although CHS programs are required to consider the availability of alternate resources when deciding whether to approve a referral, IHS officials acknowledged that programs may not always take this into consideration when making their decision.

Providers reported a number of reasons for which they received denials for payment from CHS programs. While providers said that some of the denials they received were related to patient eligibility, such as a patient living outside of the CHS delivery area, which was noted by four providers, most of the denials they received were related to administrative requirements. Twelve providers indicated that one of the most common reasons for denial was that an alternate resource was available to the patient. Other common administrative denial reasons included the availability and accessibility of IHS facilities to deliver services, noted by seven providers, and failure to provide notification within 72 hours of the patient receiving emergency services, noted by six providers. Seven providers also stated that they received denials because the CHS program determined that the care was non-emergent or not within medical priority for which funding was available. In addition, eight providers stated that some denials may have occurred because CHS patients may not have had a clear understanding of CHS policies and procedures related to payment. Eight providers stated that CHS patients could benefit from education on CHS procedures, including the need to obtain a CHS program referral prior to receiving care and the understanding that a CHS program referral does not guarantee payment.

Obtaining Payments from CHS Programs

Fourteen providers who we interviewed reported challenges obtaining timely payment from CHS programs. Seven of these providers stated that these delays occurred in obtaining a purchase order. However, six providers stated that after they obtained a purchase order from the CHS program, they received payment from IHS's fiscal intermediary in a timely manner. In fiscal year 2010, IHS reported that the average number of days between receiving a provider claim and issuing a purchase order was 82 days, 4 days more than the agency's target of 78 days for that fiscal year.[45] Of the providers who we interviewed, 12 providers stated that it has taken several months, or in some cases years, to receive payment for CHS program claims. Seven providers said that these delays tended to occur when the CHS program's funding for the fiscal year had been depleted. According to IHS officials, delays in issuing purchase orders can be attributed to several factors, including a shortage of the CHS program staff who process purchase orders and the lengthy amount of time it takes providers to send patient medical records needed to make a determination for CHS payment.

Fourteen providers stated that the CHS program's paper-based claims process required a lot of paperwork to be submitted, such as a patient's medical records, or was otherwise time consuming. Twelve providers also stated that for some payers with which they interacted, including Medicare and Medicaid, they were able to process claims electronically, which in some cases also allowed them to electronically track a claim's status. In contrast, to obtain payment for emergency care through the CHS program, providers have had to send paper copies of patient medical records and a paper claim to the CHS program to be reviewed. Seven providers stated that this process had led to delays because CHS staff may lose paperwork and then ask the provider to resubmit the information. However, seven other providers noted that they were electronically submitting claims for payment to IHS's fiscal intermediary, or working with CHS programs to begin this process, which should reduce the amount of required paperwork.[46]

Some providers also stated that it was difficult to determine the status of claims while waiting for approval to be paid. Four providers said that when they contacted CHS program staff to determine the status of claims, the staff were not always able to provide the information. Of these providers, two said that CHS programs did not communicate the status of submitted claims. Additionally, one provider told us that one federal CHS program with which they interacted did not communicate to them when a claim had been denied.[47]

Instead, the CHS program provided no response to the provider's claim for payment.[48] IHS officials acknowledged that additional agency efforts toward improving customer service are needed to ensure that CHS program staff communicate more promptly with providers.

Receiving Communications on CHS Policies and Procedures to Receive Payment

Eighteen providers noted challenges receiving communications from IHS about CHS policies and procedures related to payment, including having had few, if any, formal meetings with program staff and a lack of training and guidance. For example, 10 providers stated that they had never met CHS program staff or did not meet regularly with them, although eight other providers said that they benefited from regular communications with CHS program staff, such as establishing good working relationships with CHS program staff and getting assistance in clarifying CHS program policies and procedures to receive payments. According to the *Standards for Internal Control in the Federal Government* and the *Internal Control Management and Evaluation Tool*, agency management should ensure that there are adequate means of timely and effective communication with, and obtaining information from, external stakeholders that have significant impact on the agency achieving its goals and an agency should employ many and various means of communications, such as policy and procedure manuals and Internet web pages.[49] By not ensuring that its CHS programs have timely and effective communication with external providers about CHS policies and procedures related to payment, IHS has no reasonable assurance that the agency is achieving its objectives.

The providers who we interviewed generally indicated that their understanding of the CHS program came from experience, rather than communications, including formal training and guidance from IHS. Twelve providers stated that they had at least a basic understanding of CHS policies and procedures for obtaining CHS payments. The providers we interviewed told us that the amount of training they received from IHS varied. While 3 of 4 providers in one IHS area stated that they received recent training from the staff of CHS programs or their area office, 13 providers in other areas told us that they had never received training from IHS staff or had not received training in many years. Of those 13 providers, 6 mentioned that they had not received educational materials, including guidance, about the CHS program. Instead, 6 providers stated that their knowledge of the CHS program had been self-taught or obtained from working with CHS program staff. In contrast, 7 providers stated that other payers with which they interacted provided regular on- site training, guidance manuals, or online resources that allowed them to learn about a payer's payment policies. IHS officials said that the responsibility for educating providers is delegated to the area offices. According to IHS officials, during past meetings with area office staff, they have emphasized the importance of external provider training and shared area office best practices for educating providers. IHS headquarters officials also stated that, in 2009, they developed a CHS program manual for external providers and sent it to the area offices to be distributed to providers.[50] However, IHS officials acknowledged that, given the complexity of the CHS program, additional agency efforts are needed to ensure that all IHS areas are engaged in external provider education.[51]

In the absence of training from IHS, one provider stated that it had developed its own training on the CHS program. This provider used the experience of one of its staff members who had previously worked for the CHS program to provide training to multiple health care facilities within its health system. However, that staff member had not received any training from either individual CHS programs or the area office since being hired by the provider 4 years ago and, therefore, would not have been aware of any policy changes IHS made during that time.

Most Providers Generally Reported That CHS Program Challenges Contributed to Patient and Provider Burden

Most providers who we interviewed generally reported that challenges with the CHS program, particularly denied payment for services, added to the burden of both patients and providers. Twenty-two providers stated that when care they provided was denied by the CHS program, they billed the patient. Of these providers, 3 stated that, because of the length of time that it took the CHS program to approve or deny a service, they started billing the patient even if a denial had not yet been received.[52] For example, 1 provider stated that they used to wait as long as 4 years for CHS programs to make claims decisions, but they now bill the patient if they do not receive communication from CHS programs within a timeframe typical to that of other payers.[53]

Twelve providers told us that, for the care denied by CHS programs that was billed to patients, either they were not able to obtain payment or patients did not apply for provider payment assistance programs. Eleven providers stated that they were only able to collect a small portion of the care billed to

American Indian and Alaska Native patients or patients for whom payment was denied. Of the 12 providers who discussed how uncompensated care is classified in their financial records, all indicated that it was considered bad debt if the patient was not able to pay for services or qualify for charity care.[54] One provider estimated that it had a collections rate of about 1 percent for services billed to patients denied by the CHS program. The provider noted that while CHS patients accounted for about 30 percent of its patient population, they accounted for about 85 percent of the provider's bad debt. Ten providers stated that when the patients' bill was not paid, they were turned over to collections.[55] In addition, 18 providers had a charity care program, which offered reduced charges or free care to patients who met income and other requirements and was available to patients whose care was denied for payment by the CHS program. However, 8 of these providers stated that patients for whom CHS program payment was denied generally did not apply for charity care, and 8 of the other 10 providers did not mention or did not have information on the number of patients denied by the CHS program that applied for charity care.[56]

Providers varied in whether they reported that this uncompensated care affected their operations. Ten providers, including five of the eight critical access hospitals that we interviewed,[57] reported that the amount of uncompensated care associated with the CHS program affected them financially by, among other things, limiting their ability to purchase new equipment or resulting in increased costs to other patients. One critical access hospital stated that because of the uncompensated care associated with the CHS program, it was seeking new ownership. However, four providers who we interviewed told us that the amount of uncompensated care had not significantly affected them financially. Additionally, some providers sought payment from other resources for services delivered to patients. For example, eight providers, seven of which were larger than critical access hospitals, stated that they hired a benefits coordinator or were able to get their state health benefits agency to place a benefits coordinator at their facility to assist patients in applying for alternate resources, such as Medicaid.

The providers who we interviewed told us that these burdens had varying effects on the delivery of care to patients. Nine of the 12 providers who discussed this issue with us stated that they provided care to patients regardless of their ability to obtain payment from the CHS program. In addition, the Emergency Medical Treatment and Active Labor Act (EMTALA) requires most hospitals to provide an examination and needed stabilizing treatment, without consideration of insurance coverage or ability to pay, when a patient presents to an emergency room for attention to an emergency medical condition.[58] However, 3 of the 7 office-based providers that we interviewed said that when dealing with the CHS program, generally, they only saw patients who had obtained a CHS program referral.

CONCLUSION

IHS's CHS program serves as an important resource for American Indian and Alaska Native individuals who need health care services not available at IHS-funded federal and tribal facilities. Despite recent funding increases, most federal and tribal CHS programs that responded to our surveys reported that they did not have funds available to pay for all requested health care services for patients who otherwise met requirements, including emergent and acutely urgent care. However, IHS's estimate of the extent to which unmet need exists in the CHS program is not reliable because of deficiencies in the agency's oversight of the collection of unfunded services data on which it relies to develop this estimate. IHS's acknowledgement of these limitations and the early efforts of its workgroup to explore additional options for estimating need are positive steps. However, IHS has not yet completed the development of its new method for estimating CHS program need using the FDI or made a decision about how it will use deferral and denial data to help estimate CHS program need. Further, as its workgroup has noted, reliably captured deferral and denial data on all patients would present the strongest evidence of CHS program need. Therefore, it continues to be important that the agency take steps to ensure that complete and consistent deferral and denial data are collected. IHS has not provided adequate oversight to ensure that the annual reports it receives from each area office and uses to estimate unmet need include data from all of their federal CHS programs. In addition, although the agency cannot require reporting by tribal CHS programs, its efforts to provide outreach have not been sufficient to encourage such reporting from all tribal programs. Without complete reporting from federal and tribal programs, IHS does not have complete data for its estimate of unmet need. In addition, the agency's ability to determine the completeness of the data it collects and take steps to improve reporting is limited because its current template does not provide sufficient detail about which federal and tribal programs are reporting deferral and denial counts. As IHS responds to the future recommendations of its workgroup, the agency should ensure that it expeditiously addresses the weaknesses we identified in the deferral and denial data that provide the agency with information about program need.

Given the decentralized nature of the CHS program, effective guidance, training, and oversight by IHS can help ensure that policies and procedures affecting its determination of need are consistently applied across CHS programs. Our survey results suggest that current agency practices have not ensured consistent recording of unfunded services by CHS programs. Documenting how IHS uses unfunded services data to assess CHS program need could help ensure that area offices and CHS programs maintain data collection practices that contribute to the reliability of IHS's estimate of need.

Given that CHS program funds may be depleted before the end of the fiscal year, it is important that CHS programs take steps to maximize the care that patients receive. However, they should not engage in practices that risk incurring obligations in excess of the available funding. IHS officials acknowledge that the guidance that IHS provides to CHS program staff on funds management may not be sufficient to ensure that CHS programs do not engage in problematic funds management practices.

Effective communication with providers is an important element of IHS's oversight to ensure proper CHS program management. The providers we spoke with noted challenges related to their participation in the CHS program that they said created a burden for themselves and their patients. Among their concerns was a lack of timely and effective communication with the individual CHS programs to determine whether or when CHS programs would provide payment for services provided to American Indian and Alaska Native patients. Timely and effective communication between IHS and providers is especially important to ensuring efficient program operations. As acknowledged by IHS officials, the complexity of the CHS program makes this communication particularly important. The challenges that providers described— determining patient eligibility for payment, contacting CHS programs with questions about claims, and ensuring the timely receipt of payment— would be mitigated by improved CHS program processes and communications, including training.

RECOMMENDATIONS FOR EXECUTIVE ACTION

To develop more accurate data for estimating the funds needed for the CHS program and improving IHS oversight, we recommend that the Secretary of Health and Human Services direct the Director of IHS to take the following eight actions:

- ensure that area offices submit data on unfunded services from all federal CHS programs;
- conduct outreach and technical assistance to tribal CHS programs to encourage and support their efforts to voluntarily provide data that can be used to better estimate the needs of tribal CHS programs;
- develop an annual data reporting template that requires area offices to report available deferral and denial counts for each federal and tribal CHS program;
- develop a plan and timeline for improving the agency's deferral and denial data;
- develop written guidance, provide training, and conduct oversight activities necessary to ensure unfunded services data are consistently and completely recorded by federal CHS programs;
- develop a written policy documenting how IHS evaluates need for the CHS program and disseminate it to area offices and CHS programs to ensure they understand how unfunded services data are used to estimate overall program needs;
- provide written guidance to CHS programs on a process to use when funds are depleted and there is a continued need for services, and monitor to ensure that appropriate actions are taken; and
- develop ways to enhance CHS program communication with providers, such as providing regular trainings on patient eligibility and claim approval decisions to providers.

Agency and Tribal Comments and Our Evaluation

We provided a draft of this report to HHS for review and comment and subsequently met with HHS and IHS officials to obtain additional information. In its written comments, HHS indicated steps that IHS would take to implement some of our recommendations and discussed steps the agency was taking to implement a new method for estimating CHS program need. HHS and IHS officials subsequently provided us with clarification about the status of IHS's plans for estimating program need and HHS submitted revised written comments. HHS's letter and revised general written comments are reprinted in appendix III. We also provided tribal representatives with an opportunity to present oral comments and the representatives we spoke with primarily discussed the role of tribal programs in IHS's needs assessment process. The comments from HHS and the tribal representatives are summarized below.

In its original written comments, HHS commented that IHS is making efforts to address the problems identified in our draft report and provided additional information about the development of its new methodology for estimating program need. With regard to our first five recommendations to improve the collection of deferral and denial data from individual CHS programs, HHS agreed that these data are incomplete and inconsistent. HHS also agreed that such data could provide a reliable estimate of need if they were universally and uniformly collected. However, HHS indicated that IHS's proposed new method for estimating CHS program need by adapting its existing FDI would provide IHS with a sufficiently reliable estimate of CHS program need without relying on deferral and denial data. In our draft report, we acknowledged that IHS has taken positive steps to identify and examine the weaknesses in its current data and explore other sources of data to estimate CHS program need, such as exploring the use of the FDI method. As HHS noted in its comments, the IHS Director's Workgroup proposing this methodology has not yet issued a final recommendation to the Director of IHS for approval.

Following the receipt of HHS's original written comments, we met with HHS and IHS officials to obtain clarification about the status of IHS's plans for assessing CHS program need. The officials confirmed that the agency was continuing to develop the new method by adapting the FDI methodology to measure CHS program need. They said that the new method had not yet been formally recommended to the Director and that IHS did not have a formal agency approved plan for implementing it. IHS officials also indicated the agency had not yet determined the extent to which deferral and denial data would continue to be used by IHS headquarters to estimate program need if the FDI method is adopted. However, they indicated that until this decision is made, the agency will continue to collect deferral and denial data from the area offices.

As we noted in our draft, the FDI method would be adapted to provide IHS with an estimate of funding needed to provide care to American Indians and Alaska Natives through the CHS program at a level comparable to the care available through the health insurance program available to federal employees. IHS's Director's Workgroup previously indicated that reliably captured deferral and denial data on all patients would present the strongest evidence of CHS program need. Given that the proposed FDI methodology is still in early development and IHS plans to continue collecting deferral and denial data, we believe that expeditious implementation of our first five recommendations is vital to ensure the data IHS uses to calculate program need are accurate. With regard to our other three recommendations, HHS described in its comments the steps that IHS would take to develop a written policy on how IHS evaluates CHS program need and provide training to CHS program officials on the process to use when funds are depleted. HHS also indicated that the IHS Director's Workgroup would be providing recommendations for enhancing communication with providers. HHS also provided us with technical comments, which we incorporated as appropriate.

Subsequent to our conversation with HHS and IHS officials, HHS submitted revised comments to our report. In the revisions, HHS clarified that the FDI method represents one of multiple options for estimating unmet need that IHS's Director's Workgroup is considering and clarified that the development of this new methodology is still ongoing. The revisions HHS made to its written comments do not substantively change our response.

We also provided tribal representatives, including the 177 tribal CHS programs we surveyed and the three tribal advocacy groups we interviewed, the opportunity to provide oral comments on a draft of this report. Representatives from 11 tribal CHS programs and two tribal advocacy groups provided comments. The most frequent comment related to our recommendation that IHS provide outreach and technical assistance to tribal CHS programs to encourage them to submit data that can be used to assess CHS program need. Specifically, representatives from 2 tribal CHS programs stated that more technical assistance from IHS would be helpful, because it is important that the needs of the tribal programs be captured in IHS's needs assessment. A tribal advocacy group representative noted that some tribes have chosen not to collect deferral and denial data because of its cost burden. A representative from a tribal CHS program noted the added cost of tracking these data was justified by the benefit they provide to IHS's budget process. In addition, a tribal representative expressed concern that our finding on the accuracy of IHS's estimate of need could be interpreted to suggest that the actual level of need is lower than what IHS is estimating. In our report, we did not examine whether or not IHS's estimate of need over- or under-estimates the actual level of unfunded need, but rather found that the estimate is not reliable because of deficiencies in the agency's oversight of the collection of unfunded services data.

We are sending copies of this report to the Secretary of Health and Human Services and other interested parties. In addition, the report is available at no charge on the GAO web site at http://www.gao.gov.

If you or your staffs have any questions about this report, please contact me at (202) 512-7114 or kingk@gao.gov. Contact points for our Offices of Congressional Relations and Public Affairs may be found on the last page of this report. GAO staff who made major contributions to this report are listed in appendix IV.

Kathleen M. King
Director, Health Care

List of Addressees

The Honorable Daniel Akaka
Chairman
The Honorable John Barrasso
Ranking Member
Committee on Indian Affairs
United States Senate

The Honorable Don Young
Chairman
The Honorable Dan Boren
Ranking Member
Subcommittee on Indian and Alaska Native Affairs
Committee on Natural Resources
House of Representatives

Jeff Bingaman
Tim Johnson
Lisa Murkowski
John Thune
United States Senate

APPENDIX I: SCOPE AND METHODOLOGY

In this report, we examined (1) the extent to which the Indian Health Service (IHS) ensures the data it collects on unfunded services are accurate to determine a reliable estimate of contract health services (CHS) program need, (2) the extent to which federal and tribal CHS programs report having funds available to pay for contract health services, and (3) the experiences of external providers in obtaining payment from the CHS program.

To address part of our work for our first two objectives, we administered two surveys—one each to federal and tribal CHS programs. From March 2010 through August 2010, we obtained lists of federal and tribal CHS programs from each area office, from which we identified 66 federal CHS programs and 177 tribal CHS programs. We administered a web-based survey to all of the federal CHS programs from October 2010 through January 2011. In addition, from September 2010 through January 2011, we administered a mixed-mode survey—both web-based and by mail—to all of the tribal CHS programs; this survey was blinded to maintain the anonymity of respondents. To ensure the clarity and precision of our survey questions, we pretested our federal CHS program survey with officials from IHS and our tribal CHS program survey with officials from three tribal health advocacy groups and a tribal health official. We analyzed complete survey data from all 66 federal CHS programs, for a response rate of 100 percent, and 103 of 177 tribal CHS programs, for a response rate of 58 percent.[59] The results from our survey of tribal CHS programs are not generalizable to all tribal CHS programs because we did not receive responses from all tribal CHS programs and tribal programs vary due to the flexibility tribes have in administering their programs. We relied on the data as reported by the CHS program officials who were identified as the primary contacts for the CHS program and did not independently verify these data or ask IHS to verify them. However, we reviewed all responses for reasonableness and internal consistency. For our survey of federal CHS programs, when necessary, we followed up with the program officials who completed our survey for clarification.

Based on these activities, we determined these data were sufficiently reliable for the purpose of our report.

We also conducted site visits to IHS area offices based in Oklahoma City, Oklahoma and Portland, Oregon in March and April, 2010. During these site visits, we interviewed area office officials and representatives from a total of four federal and eight tribal CHS programs located in those areas. In addition, we interviewed officials from IHS headquarters and each of IHS's 12 area offices to discuss oversight of the CHS program, and spoke with three tribal health advocacy groups. We also examined IHS oversight, such as the provision of policy and guidance, conducted to ensure that CHS programs consistently and completely record and report unfunded services data. We compared these oversight activities to the standards described in the *Standards for Internal Control in the Federal Government* and the *Internal Control Management and Evaluation Tool.*[60] We also reviewed our cost estimating guide to assess procedures for determining a reliable estimate for budgetary purposes.[61]

To examine the experiences of external providers in obtaining payment from the CHS program, we interviewed representatives from hospitals and office-based health care providers from selected IHS areas. We selected four areas from which to identify providers based on their fiscal year 2009 per capita CHS program funding and dependency on CHS funds for hospital services. We estimated per capita funding using the agency's fiscal year 2009 user population estimates and allocation of CHS program funds.[62] To estimate dependency, we used an IHS measure of dependency it uses to allocate certain funds to the area offices. It measures whether patients in an area have practical access to IHS-funded federally and tribally operated hospitals.[63] If the patients do not have access to such facilities, then they are considered to be more dependent on the CHS program for hospital services and therefore, the area receives additional funding. The four areas we selected were Bemidji, Billings, Phoenix, and Oklahoma City,[64] which represent areas that were above or below average for each of our selection criteria. (See table 3.) In fiscal year 2009, the four areas represented 43 percent of the IHS user population and received 37 percent of CHS funding.

Within these four areas, we selected 23 providers—16 hospitals and 7 office-based providers—to interview. Most of these providers were identified through our survey of federal CHS programs as providers who provided the highest volume of care to CHS program users in fiscal year 2009. In addition, we also identified providers who interact frequently with CHS programs through our discussions with state hospital associations and a tribal health advocacy group. Given the small number of providers in our sample and our process for selecting them, the results from these interviews are not generalizable to all providers interacting with the CHS program. We asked providers about their experiences obtaining effective and timely communication related to the payment process, such as training or guidance on determining patient eligibility for CHS program payment of services and determining the status of claims, and compared their experiences with the standards described in the *Standards for Internal Control in the Federal Government* and the *Internal Control Management and Evaluation Tool.*[65] We asked providers a standard set of open-ended questions and we did not independently validate their reported experiences, but we did discuss many of their comments with IHS officials.

We conducted this performance audit from January 2010 to September 2011 in accordance with generally accepted government auditing standards. Those standards require that we plan and perform the audit to obtain sufficient, appropriate evidence to provide a reasonable basis for our findings and conclusions based on our audit objectives. We believe that the evidence obtained provides a reasonable basis for our findings and conclusions based on our audit objectives.

Table 2. Categorization of Area Offices by Selection Criteria

Category	Area office	Per capita CHS program funding in fiscal year 2009	Percent of CHS-dependent operating units in fiscal year 2009[a]
Above average funding, above average CHS dependency	Bemidji	$407.35	94.1%
	Nashville	$470.84	92.0%
	Portland	$664.30	100.0%
	California	$399.34	100.0%
Above average funding, below average CHS dependency	Billings	$694.50	62.5%
	Tucson	$579.21	50.0%
	Aberdeen	$557.27	59.1%
	Alaska	$456.01	15.8%
Below average funding, above average CHS dependency	Phoenix	$323.90	72.7%
Below average funding, below average CHS dependency	Oklahoma City	$237.61	32.0%
	Navajo	$286.54	16.7%
	Albuquerque	$347.09	50.0%
Average		**$392.19**	**71.9%**

Source: GAO analysis of IHS documents.

[a] Operating units are the entities at the local level that have financial responsibility for CHS-eligible persons.

Appendix II: Catastrophic Health Emergency Fund

The Indian Health Care Amendments of 1988 established the Catastrophic Health Emergency Fund (CHEF) to meet the medical costs associated with treating catastrophic illnesses or victims of disasters.[66] CHEF is administered centrally within the Indian Health Service (IHS) and reimburses federal and tribal contract health services (CHS) programs on a first-come first-served basis for CHS program cases with costs exceeding the threshold set annually within the range established by law.[67] Specifically, CHS programs pay for the services and then request reimbursement from IHS for expenses over the threshold, which was $25,000 in fiscal year 2009.[68] In fiscal year 2009, IHS reimbursed 1,223 cases at a total cost of $31 million; in fiscal year 2010, IHS reimbursed 1,747 cases at a total cost of $48 million. The top three diagnostic categories funded in fiscal year 2010 were injuries, cancer, and heart disease.

When CHEF funds are depleted, requests for reimbursement are denied by IHS. As part of IHS's needs assessment for the CHS program, the agency determines the number of CHEF requests for reimbursement that were denied and then uses the actual billed charges that were submitted by CHS programs to determine the cost of these services. In fiscal year 2009, IHS denied 1,065 cases totaling $24 million; in fiscal year 2010, it denied 865 cases totaling $14 million. However, IHS speculated that this may underestimate the need for CHEF reimbursement because additional cases may have qualified for CHEF reimbursement, but CHS programs may not have submitted a request for reimbursement due to the depletion of CHEF before the end of the fiscal year.

CHEF Survey Data: Federal CHS Programs

Of the 66 federal CHS programs we surveyed, 52 reported that they submitted requests for CHEF reimbursement in fiscal year 2009. Of these, 12 reported that they did not continue to submit requests for CHEF reimbursement once the CHS program learned that CHEF funds were depleted. Of the 66 federal CHS programs we surveyed, 14 reported that they did not submit any requests for CHEF reimbursement in fiscal year 2009. The most common reasons they reported for not submitting requests for CHEF reimbursement were that the CHS program did not experience any cases costing over $25,000 (8 of 14 federal CHS programs) and staffing shortages (5 of 14 federal CHS programs).

CHEF Survey Data: Tribal CHS Programs

Of the 103 tribal CHS programs who responded to our survey, 46 submitted requests for CHEF reimbursement in fiscal year 2009. Fifty-three of the tribal CHS programs reported that they did not submit requests for CHEF reimbursement. The most common reasons they reported for not submitting requests for CHEF reimbursement were that the CHS program did not experience any cases costing over $25,000 (31 of 53 tribal CHS programs) and tribal programs were unable to pay for the first $25,000 of expenses (13 of 53 tribal CHS programs).

APPENDIX III: COMMENTS FROM THE DEPARTMENT OF HEALTH AND HUMAN SERVICES

DEPARTMENT OF HEALTH & HUMAN SERVICES   OFFICE OF THE SECRETARY

Assistant Secretary for Legislation
Washington, DC 20201

Kathleen M. King, Director
Health Care
U.S. Government Accountability Office
441 G Street NW
Washington, DC 20548

SEP 19 2011

Dear Ms. King:

Attached are comments on the U.S. Government Accountability Office's (GAO) draft report entitled, "INDIAN HEALTH SERVICE: Increased Oversight Needed to Ensure Accuracy of Data Used for Estimating Contract Health Service Need" (GAO-11-767).

The Department appreciates the opportunity to review this report before its publication.

Sincerely,

Jim R. Esquea
Assistant Secretary for Legislation

Attachment

GENERAL COMMENTS OF THE DEPARTMENT OF HEALTH AND HUMAN SERVICES (HHS) ON THE GOVERNMENT ACCOUNTABILITY OFFICE'S (GAO) DRAFT REPORT ENTITLED, "INDIAN HEALTH SERVICE: INCREASED OVERSIGHT NEEDED TO ENSURE ACCURACY OF DATA USED FOR ESTIMATING CONTRACT HEALTH SERVICE NEED" (GAO-11-767)

The Department appreciates the opportunity to review and comment on this draft report. The Indian Health Service (IHS) acknowledges that oversight activities related to the identification of Contract Health Service (CHS) unmet need estimates have not been carried out to the extent described in the GAO's Standards for Internal Control in the Federal Government.

Procedures described and reviewed during this engagement reflect IHS' response to questions regarding the estimated additional dollar amount needed to fund all Priority I cases (the unmet need). As cited in the report, the IHS has established a workgroup to evaluate methods to quantify the need due to increased interest in CHS program unmet need. The IHS will establish appropriate management controls once the CHS workgroup recommendation for the methodology for determining CHS unmet need is finalized.

The report states that data that IHS collected from CHS programs were incomplete and inconsistent. It concludes that "a reliable estimate of need will require complete and consistent data from each of the individual CHS programs." We agree that reporting has been incomplete and inconsistent. We agree that additional funds needed for CHS could be reliably calculated if all denied or deferred cases were universally and uniformly reported. We believe that sufficiently reliable estimates of CHS funding needs may also be calculated using methods and data that are independent of denial and deferral counts reported by individual CHS programs.

The CHS workgroup is reviewing several options for estimating the CHS need. One option under discussion that can estimate the need with reasonable, although not absolute assurance, is the Federal Disparity Index (FDI) method which is used by the IHS already to estimate resource needs for the IHS user population. The FDI based alternative approach to calculating needs is referenced on page 21-23 of your report. The FDI method can be adapted to calculate CHS resources as a sub-set of total needed health care resources. Such estimates are sufficiently reliable for annual CHS budget requests and other purposes. Adapting the FDI method for this purpose will not impose significant new data collection burdens.

GAO Recommendations

To develop more accurate data for estimating the funds needed for the CHS program and improving IHS oversight, we recommend that the Secretary of Health and Human Services direct the Director of IHS to take the following eight actions:

- *ensure that area offices submit data on unfunded services from all federal CHS programs;*
- *conduct outreach and technical assistance to tribal CHS programs to encourage and support their efforts to voluntarily provide data that can be used to better estimate the needs of tribal CHs programs;*
- *develop an annual data reporting template that requires area offices to report available deferral and denial counts for each federal and tribal CHS program;*
- *develop a plan and timeline for improving the agency's deferral and denial data;*

GENERAL COMMENTS OF THE DEPARTMENT OF HEALTH AND HUMAN SERVICES (HHS) ON THE GOVERNMENT ACCOUNTABILITY OFFICE'S (GAO) DRAFT REPORT ENTITLED, "INDIAN HEALTH SERVICE: INCREASED OVERSIGHT NEEDED TO ENSURE ACCURACY OF DATA USED FOR ESTIMATING CONTRACT HEALTH SERVICE NEED" (GAO-11-767)

- *develop written guidance, provide training, and conduct oversight activities necessary to ensure unfunded services data are consistently and completely recorded by federal CHS programs;*
- *develop a written policy documenting how IHS evaluates need for the CHS program and disseminate it to area offices and CHS programs to ensure they understand how unfunded services data are used to estimate overall program needs;*
- *provide written guidance to CHS programs on a process to use when funds are depleted and there is a continued need for services, and monitor to ensure that appropriate actions are taken; and*
- *develop ways to enhance CHS program communication with providers, such as providing regular trainings on patient eligibility and claim approval decision to providers.*

Concerning the first five recommendations, the CHS workgroup is discussing options for estimating unmet need and are conducting a pilot study of one such option. The workgroup will review the pilot study and make recommendations to the IHS Director.

In response to the last three recommendations, we offer the following comments:

- The IHS will develop a written policy on how IHS evaluates CHS need and disseminate it to Area offices to ensure they understand how unfunded services data are used to estimate CHS need. This will be accomplished after the Director has approved the method for estimating CHS need.

- The IHS currently has a policy on the process to use when funds are depleted and there is a continued need for services which will be provided to all CHS program Officers. CHS program officers will provide training on the Agency's policy regarding use of funds.

- The IHS has developed a provider training manual for use in educating providers on CHS patient eligibility and claim approval processes. The Directors Workgroup on Improving CHS will provide recommendations for improving and enhancing CHS program communication with providers.

APPENDIX IV: STAFF ACKNOWLEDGMENTS

Staff Acknowledgments

In addition to the contact names above, Catina Bradley, Martha Kelly, and Suzanne Worth, Assistant Directors; George Bogart; Zhi Boon; William Hadley; Giselle Hicks; Darryl Joyce; Hannah Locke; Sarah-Lynn McGrath; Jasleen Modi; Lisa Motley; Laurie Pachter; and Mario Ramsey made key contributions to this report.

End Notes

[1] See, for example, GAO, *Indian Health Service: Basic Services Mostly Available; Substance Abuse Problems Need Attention,* GAO/HRD-93-48 (Washington, D.C.: Apr. 9, 1993); and *U.S. Commission on Civil Rights, Broken Promises: Evaluating the Native American Health Care System* (Washington, D.C.: September 2004).

[2] IHS defines an Indian tribe as any Indian tribe, band, nation, group, Pueblo, or community, including any Alaska Native village or Native group, which is federally recognized as eligible for the programs and services provided by the United States to Indians because of their status as Indians.

[3] Under the Indian Self-Determination and Education Assistance Act, as amended, federally recognized Indian tribes can enter into self-determination contracts or self- governance compacts with the Secretary of Health and Human Services to take over administration of IHS programs for Indians previously administered by IHS on their behalf. Self-governance compacts allow tribes to consolidate and assume administration of all programs, services, activities, and competitive grants administered throughout IHS, or portions thereof, that are carried out for the benefit of Indians because of their status as Indians. In contrast, self determination contracts allow tribes to assume administration of a program, programs, or portions thereof. See 25 U.S.C. §§ 450f(a) (self determination contracts), 458aaa-4(b)(1) (self-governance compacts).

[4] IHS's 12 area offices are: Aberdeen, Alaska, Albuquerque, Bemidji, Billings, California, Nashville, Navajo, Oklahoma City, Phoenix, Portland, and Tucson.

[5] GAO, *Indian Health Service: Health Care Services Are Not Always Available to Native Americans,* GAO-05-789 (Washington, D.C.: Aug. 31, 2005).

[6] In fiscal year 2008, IHS received about $579 million for the CHS program.

[7] This work originated as a request from the Senate Committee on Indian Affairs and individual members prior to the enactment of the Patient Protection and Affordable Care Act, which provided for the enactment of the Indian Health Care Improvement Reauthorization and Extension Act of 2009. The act also requires GAO to complete other work on aspects of the CHS program, including funds distribution and claims payment. See Pub. L. No. 111-148, § 10221, 124 Stat. 119, 935 (2010) (enacting S. 1790, as reported by the Committee on Indian Affairs in the Senate in December 2009, into law with amendments); S. 1790, 111th Cong. §§ 137, 199 (2009).

[8] GAO, *Standards for Internal Control in the Federal Government,* GAO/AIMD-00-21 .3.1 (Washington, D.C.: November 1999); and *Internal Control Management and Evaluation Tool,* GAO-01-1008G (Washington, D.C.: August 2001). Internal control is synonymous with management control and comprises the plans, methods, and procedures used to meet missions, goals, and objectives.

[9] GAO, *GAO Cost Estimating and Assessment Guide: Best Practices for Developing and Managing Capital Program Costs,* GAO-09-3SP (Washington, D.C.: March 2009).

[10] We measured dependency using an IHS measure of patient access to an IHS-funded hospital. Patients in some areas do not have access to an IHS-funded hospital. Therefore, IHS distributes additional CHS funds to such areas, because patients in these locations are more dependent on the CHS program to receive hospital-based services.

[11] The Bemidji area includes locations in Indiana, Minnesota, Michigan, and Wisconsin; the Billings area includes locations in Montana and Wyoming; the Phoenix area includes locations in Arizona, California, Nevada, and Utah; and the Oklahoma City area includes locations in Oklahoma, Kansas, and Texas.

[12] GAO/AIMD-00-21.3.1 and GAO-01-1008G.

[13] Most CHS program funds are allocated according to historical funding levels that are typically adjusted annually for inflation and population growth.

[14] Tribal CHS programs are able to supplement their CHS program funds received from IHS with reimbursements from Medicare, Medicaid, and private insurance for services provided at their tribal health care facilities. Tribal CHS programs are also able to supplement their CHS funding with tribal funds earned from tribal business or enterprises. See 25 U.S.C. § 1621f.

[15] Medicaid is a jointly funded federal-state health care program that covers certain low- income individuals and families. Medicare is the federal government's health care insurance program for individuals aged 65 and older and for individuals with certain disabilities or end-stage renal disease.

[16] See 25 U.S.C. §§ 1621e, 1623; 42 C.F.R. § 136.61 (2010). There are certain exemptions to the CHS program's designation as a payer of last resort. For example, certain tribally funded insurance plans are not considered alternate resources and the CHS program must pay for care before billing the tribally funded insurance plan. The CHS program must also pay for care provided to eligible American Indians and Alaska Natives before the crime victim compensation program, a federal program that provides compensation to victims and survivors of criminal violence.

[17] IHS contracts with BlueCross BlueShield of New Mexico to serve as its fiscal intermediary to validate and pay all federal CHS program claims.

[18] Before submitting a claim for payment to the CHS program, IHS expects the external provider to seek reimbursement from any alternate resources available to the patient.

[19] Deferrals may be authorized later if additional funds become available. IHS policy requires that deferred services be for elective care, rather than emergent or urgent care. Programs may not defer payment for services already rendered, only for services that have not been received.

[20] The eight categories of denial are: (1) eligible but care not within medical priority, (2) eligible but alternate resource available, (3) patient ineligible for CHS, (4) emergency notification not within 72 hours, (5) non-emergency prior approval not authorized, (6) patient resides outside CHS delivery area, (7) IHS facility available and accessible, and (8) all other denials.

[21] CHEF was established by the Indian Health Care Amendments of 1988 to meet the medical costs associated with treating catastrophic illnesses or victims of disasters. See 25 U.S.C. §1621a.

[22] IHS headquarters officials told us they obtain these data through the annual request because they do not have the capability to directly access the CHS programs' data through the Resource and Patient Management System, an information technology system that CHS programs can use to record approved, deferred, and denied requests for contract health services or claims for payment. In addition, the individual CHS programs are not required to use the system to record data on unfunded services and some programs reported to us that they did not use the system to record either deferrals or denials.

[23] Overall, 49 of the 103 tribal CHS programs that responded to our survey reported collecting data on unfunded services. Forty-four tribal CHS programs did not collect data, with the two most common reasons reported being staffing shortages (17) and technology limitations (14). The remaining tribal CHS programs did not provide a response or did not wish to share this information.

[24] GAO/AIMD-00-21 .3.1 and GAO-01-1008G.

[25] Further, we found that IHS's fiscal year 2009 estimate of need included deferral and denial data from areas that only contained tribal CHS programs (California and Alaska). Of the 32,309 denials for "care not within medical priority" reported by the 12 area offices in fiscal year 2009 that IHS used in its needs estimate, about 10 percent were reported by the Alaska and California area offices.

[26] IHS distributed guidance that updated its definition for the denial reason "care not within medical priority" while our federal survey was being fielded. Specifically, the definition was changed from "The medical care you received is not within the CHS medical priorities.

Medical priorities must be established when funding is limited" to "CHS is limited to services that are medically indicated and within the established IHS Medical Priorities. The medical service(s) you were provided did not fall within these priorities based on the medical information received and reviewed by the IHS medical provider. Therefore, your request for payment of these services is not approved." IHS indicated that this change did not affect the way denials are categorized by CHS programs and it did not affect how the agency uses these denials in its needs assessment.

[27] The annual request sent to the area offices asks for them to report both deferral and denial data and indicates "the data and information on Deferred Services, Denials, and CHS information from these reports will be used to support unmet CHS financial needs and in preparing budget justifications for the CHS program."

[28] GAO/AIMD-00-21 .3.1.

[29] According to our surveys, 16 of the 66 federal CHS programs and 21 of the 49 tribal CHS programs that reported collecting data on unfunded services indicated that patients may be discouraged from presenting for care if they believe funds are not available to pay for services. In addition, 22 of the 66 federal CHS programs and 20 of the 49 tribal CHS programs reported that providers may choose not to write referrals when they feel it is unlikely for CHS funds to pay for services for a patient.

[30] IHS officials told us that tribal funds used to supplement CHS funding should be a part of an estimate of CHS program unmet need because tribes should not be expected to use their own funds to pay for contract health services given the federal obligation to pay for health care for eligible American Indians and Alaska Natives. In addition, they noted that not all tribes have the means to contribute financially to their CHS programs.

[31] IHS established the Director's Workgroup on Improving the CHS Program in March 2010, and charged it with reviewing tribal input to improve the CHS program, evaluating the existing formula for distributing CHS funds, and recommending improvements in the way CHS business operations are conducted within IHS and the Indian health system. Following an October 2010 meeting, the Workgroup made several recommendations to the Director, including the creation of a subcommittee to examine need in the CHS program.

[32] The FDI was developed by a joint tribal-IHS workgroup that met to determine the level of funding needed to provide all health care services—direct care through IHS-funded federal and tribal facilities and specialty health care through federally or tribally administered CHS programs—to American Indians and Alaska Natives at a level that is comparable to the nationwide FEHBP health insurance program available to federal employees. IHS has used the FDI to distribute health care funds received to carry out the Indian Health Care Improvement Act to the area offices.

[33] The remaining six programs reported having CHS funds available to pay for all services in fiscal year 2009. One of these CHS programs, for example, reported that it was unique because it only served students attending a boarding school. These six programs were located in five different IHS areas, each of which also had federal CHS programs that reported that they did not have funds available to pay for all services in that year.

[34] For example, CHS programs may budget their funding on a weekly basis.

[35] We grouped survey responses into categories of services. For example, the category of dental services includes orthodontics and prosthodontics; orthopedic services includes joint replacements and other orthopedic surgeries; vision services includes ophthalmology and optometry; and diagnostic and imaging services includes MRIs, CT scans, and X- rays.

[36] Appropriations to IHS for contract health services are apportioned by the Office of Management and Budget, allotted to area office directors, and further distributed through allowances to federal CHS programs or payments to tribal CHS programs.

[37] To help ensure compliance with the Antideficiency Act, which generally prohibits federal officers and employees from incurring obligations in excess of appropriations, apportionments, and certain administrative subdivisions of funds, IHS has promulgated a funds management policy. See 31 U.S.C. §§ 1341, 1514, 1517. The existing policy provides

that, even if there is no violation of the Antideficiency Act, agency officials may be subject to administrative discipline should they incur obligations in excess of the funds distributed to them. *See Indian Health Manual, Circular 95-19, Administrative Control of Funds Policy; Indian Health Manual, Circular 91-7, Contract Health Service Funds Control.* IHS officials told us that the *Indian Health Manual* needs to be updated to reflect current procedures for the administrative subdivision of funds, among other things, but that the agency does not consider the over-obligation of allowances to be a violation of the Antideficiency Act unless it results in an over-obligation of the related allotment.

38 An evaluation of individual programs' compliance with statutes and policies regarding the obligation of funds and funds management was outside the scope of our review. We have referred these matters to the Department of Health and Human Services Office of Inspector General (OIG) for a review and appropriate action. Given GAO's responsibilities in this area, we will remain available to provide OIG with technical assistance.

39 Of these 73 tribal CHS programs, 47 reported depleting their CHS funds before the end of the fiscal year and 26 reported they had CHS funds available to pay for at least some care all year by budgeting weekly, monthly, or quarterly.

40 We grouped survey responses into categories of services. For example, the category of dental services includes orthodontics and prosthodontics; orthopedic services includes joint replacements and other orthopedic surgeries; prescription drugs includes trial drugs and pain medications; diagnostic and imaging services includes MRIs, CT scans, and X- rays; and hospital services includes inpatient and emergency room services.

41 Unlike federal CHS programs, tribal CHS programs can use funds from tribal enterprises and reimbursements from third party health care payers such as Medicare or private insurance to supplement CHS funds. Federal CHS programs are authorized to receive reimbursements from third party health care payers, but these funds offset rather than supplement IHS funding. See 25 U.S.C. § 1621f.

42 Since the Patient Protection and Affordable Care Act provided for the enactment of the Indian Health Care Improvement Reauthorization and Extension Act of 2009, waivers are no longer needed and tribal CHS programs are explicitly authorized to use CHS funds from IHS to purchase private insurance. See 25 U.S.C. § 1642 (amended by Pub. L. No. 111-148, § 10221, 124 Stat. 119, 935 (2010) (enacting S. 1790, 111th Cong. § 152 (2009))).

43 When a physician at an IHS-funded facility gives a referral to a patient, a copy of the referral is also sent to the CHS program committee. While a referral must be reviewed and approved by the CHS committee prior to payment, IHS officials stated that, in some instances, a patient may present for care at an external provider without first obtaining approval from the CHS program. Officials noted that it is generally indicated on the referral if it has not yet been approved.

44 The CHS program requires that if there are other health care resources available to a patient, such as Medicaid, these resources must pay for services before the CHS program because the CHS program is generally the payer of last resort. Three providers suggested that the CHS program could play a greater role in ensuring that patients are enrolled in any alternate resources prior to care being delivered. IHS's *Indian Health Manual* states that both the CHS program and providers have a responsibility to determine whether a patient would be eligible for alternate resources. IHS officials noted that provisions in the Patient Protection and Affordable Care Act could expand the availability of alternate resources for patients whose services would otherwise have been eligible for CHS program payment. In IHS's fiscal year 2012 congressional budget justification, the agency acknowledged the need to improve patients' understanding of alternate resource enrollment and assist patients with enrollment in state and federal programs and proposed new staff positions to accomplish this. IHS anticipates that enrolling patients in alternate resources will increase the availability of CHS program funds for patients without alternate resources and improve customer satisfaction.

[45] After a purchase order is issued, the provider must submit a claim to IHS's fiscal intermediary, which has a contract standard to process payment to the provider within 21 calendar days of receiving a claim.

[46] According to IHS, all providers have the option to electronically submit claims to IHS's fiscal intermediary.

[47] CHS program guidelines state that if a service received by a patient is denied CHS payment, both the patient and the provider must be notified in writing of the denial with a statement containing all the reasons for the denial.

[48] Under section 220 of the Indian Health Care Improvement Act, IHS is required to respond to a notification of a claim by a provider with either a purchase order or a denial within 5 working days after the receipt of such notification. If IHS fails to do so, it must accept the claim as valid. See 25 U.S.C. § 162 1s. Examining compliance with this requirement was beyond the scope of this review.

[49] GAO/AIMD-00-21 .3.1 and GAO-01-1008G.

[50] IHS headquarters officials said that the provider manual is not available online and providers are only able to obtain a copy if it was distributed to them through the area office.

[51] From 2006 through 2010, IHS annually conducted a national training event for CHS program staff. Some of these events have included training on customer service and educating providers. IHS's Director's Workgroup on Improving the Contract Health Services Program recently identified provider education as an important issue and recommended that IHS make provider education a nationwide initiative and develop national tools. However, IHS officials told us that the agency has not yet developed a plan to implement this recommendation.

[52] In 2005, we found that 10 of the 15 external providers that we interviewed reported that denials for or delays in payment resulted in some of the providers terminating their relationship with IHS. We noted that the termination of these relationships may affect a patient's access to care.

[53] IHS officials told us that providers should not be billing patients who are eligible for the CHS program. Under section 222 of the Indian Health Care Improvement Act, as amended by the Indian Health Care Improvement Reauthorization and Extension Act of 2009 on March 23, 2010, IHS is required to formally notify providers not later than 5 business days after receipt of notification of a claim that patients who receive authorized contract health services are not liable for any costs. See 25 U.S.C. § 1621u (amended by Pub. L. No. 111-148, § 10221, 124 Stat. 119, 935 (2010) (enacting S. 1790, 111th Cong. § 135 (2009))). IHS officials told us that this requirement is important because they heard from patients that they were being billed for services while they were waiting for the CHS program to reimburse the providers. Officials noted, however, that the requirement to send out these notifications has created a burden for CHS program staff.

[54] Bad debt is generally defined as the uncollectible payment that the patient is expected to, but does not, pay.

[55] Tribes and tribal organizations have testified before congressional committees about some of the consequences of a patient being billed for services denied by the CHS program, including negative effects on the patient's credit history and providers discontinuing services to patients because of nonpayment for services delivered.

[56] Two of the external providers that we interviewed did not have an application process associated with their charity care program.

[57] Critical access hospitals are limited to 25 beds and primarily operate in rural areas.

[58] See generally 42 U.S.C. § 1395dd.

[59] In the case of one analysis of survey data, the federal and tribal surveys asked the respective respondents to provide the three most common health care services that were (1) deferred or denied by federal CHS programs in fiscal year 2009, (2) requested but not funded by tribal CHS programs in fiscal year 2009, and (3) purchased by tribal CHS programs with tribal funds in fiscal year 2009. In our analysis of these data, we grouped the specific reported

health care services into categories of health care services for the purposes of reporting the data.

[60] GAO/AIMD-00-21.3.1 and GAO-01-1008G. Internal control is synonymous with management control and comprises the plans, methods, and procedures used to meet missions, goals, and objectives.

[61] GAO-09-3SP.

[62] According to IHS officials, the agency does not have an estimate of the number of individuals eligible to have their care paid by the CHS program. Therefore, it utilizes a user population estimate that generally represents the count of American Indian and Alaska Native individuals who had at least one direct care or contract health service inpatient stay, ambulatory care visit, or dental visit in the last 3 years.

[63] According to IHS officials, the agency considers an area to have practical access to a hospital if the hospital maintains a census of more than five patients per day and is less than 90 minutes travel time for most residents of the area.

[64] The Bemidji area includes locations in Indiana, Minnesota, Michigan, and Wisconsin; the Billings area includes locations in Montana and Wyoming; the Phoenix area includes locations in Arizona, California, Nevada, and Utah; and the Oklahoma City area includes locations in Oklahoma, Kansas, and Texas.

[65] GAO/AIMD-00-2 1.3.1 and GAO-01-1008G.

[66] See 25 U.S.C. § 1621a.

[67] The Indian Health Care Improvement Reauthorization and Extension Act of 2009, enacted by the Patient Protection and Affordable Care Act in March 2010, provided for IHS to set the threshold at $19,000, to be increased each year by a percentage established using a specific formula. See S. 1790, § 122, 111th Cong. 2009 (enacted by Pub. L. No. 111-148, § 10221, 124 Stat. 119, 935 (2010)).

[68] In certain circumstances, CHS programs can submit medical bills below the threshold to IHS and then be reimbursed on an ongoing basis at 50 percent of expenses until the completion of the case.

Chapter Sources

Chapter 1 - This is an edited, reformatted and augmented version of a Congressional Research Service publication, R41152, dated October 9, 2008.

Chapter 2 - This is an edited, reformatted and augmented version of a Congressional Research Service publication, R41630, dated February 10, 2011.

Chapter 3 - This is an edited, reformatted and augmented version of a Congressional Research Service report, GAO-11-767, dated September, 2011.

INDEX

D

E

F